Mending the S.E.A.M.:
A Process for Enhancing Traditional Depression Therapies

SI

Distributed by Seurat Innovations, LLC
www.seuratinnovations.com

A Companion Company of Lucius Seneca Wellness Group, Inc.
www.LuciusSenecaWG.org

Todd G. Kruder
Captain   USN

Dedication

To my loving wife and family.

And

To those Active Duty Military, Veterans, and their families who suffer the debilitating effects of depression.

Author's Note

The places, events, and people contained in this book are based on my recollection of them, to the best of memory's ability.

Table of Contents

Ode to Lucius Annaeus Seneca

Like the root of a tree bulging from the earthen soil below, my vein protrudes.
Where do you go my precious vein? What thrives in those channels blue?
The bluish hue reveals itself through my pail white flesh.
Where do you go my precious vein? What thrives in those channels blue?
They have been with me since birth, ignited by the spark of life itself.
Where do you go my precious vein? What thrives in those channels blue?
Without you I will certainly die. You and I will cease to exist.
Where do you go my precious vein? What thrives in those channels blue?
My mere existence is only a matter for this world. I will matter no more.
Where do you go my precious vein? What thrives in those channels blue?
With my hand I decide my very fate. Freedom is not found here.
Where do you go my precious vein? What thrives in those channels blue?
Where do you go? You pulse through my body so that I may live.
What thrives within you, my vein? My freedom.
I decide my fate this day. Today I reject those emotions telling me to do otherwise.
Lucius, today, I choose to live.

Preface

When I completed the first book, A Journey in the Fog: A Military Officer's Experience, it dawned on me; "Why not describe the process I used in more detail so others who are suffering from the effects of depression could have the same benefit?" I also realized the very same method I used, "the Waypoints", could be used in the development of the next two books in the Journey series. Trained as a Navigator, it was only natural to describe my life experiences in the context of a waypoint. I read a good definition recently that may help those less familiar with the term, "Waypoints are sets of coordinates that identify a point in physical space." Isn't that interesting? A "point in physical space". How better to describe an event in one's life than as a point in space and time. I find it humorous that the process method I'll soon be describing here, has roots in just a few paragraphs I was considering not even putting it into the first book. For those unfamiliar with my reference to the first book, allow me to summarize.

A waypoint I scribbled down one afternoon had to do with the Post-Impressionist painter (and draftsman by trade), Georges Seurat. The waypoint was labeled simply, "Seurat Dots."

Growing up in the suburbs of Chicago, one particular channel ran an infomercial spot. This particular commercial was on the subject of Georges Seurat's painting called, "A Sunday Afternoon on the Island of La Grande Jatte". The specific commercial focused on the uniqueness of this particular painting. Seurat used tiny juxtaposed dots of multi-colored paint that allowed your eye to blend colors optically, rather than having the colors physically blended on the canvas. These juxtaposed dots were referred to as, "Seurat Dots."

At this point in my writing, I had given a lot of thought to the various life experiences I felt contributed to my depression. I found it too easy to simply think my depression was rooted solely to one event or situation. I wasn't buying into anyone suggesting my depression was related to Post Traumatic Stress Disorder (PTSD). This diagnosis in my mind was a diagnosis reserved for the REAL heroes of war, not me. I contemplated, reflected, and thought through my life. I replayed those times that for whatever reason remained in the back of my mind. Those moments, when triggered by a sight, sound, situation, or even a person I might see, carried me deeper into the fog of my depression. I started to describe those instances in time. I soon discovered, I would describe them within the context of similar elements or variables. I could find elements within each "waypoint" that seemed consistent or common. In other words, I began to see a structure being formed, a diagram of sorts, and a recipe fitting for defining a process.

It dawned on me, these things I call waypoints. They could also be thought of as Seurat's Dots. Instead of colorful painted dots on a canvas, they are my experiences, one on top of the other, and one after another in time. Unlike the canvas Seurat used, these dots occur on our own canvas of our lives.

Consider your own life for just a moment. Think about those events that you experienced. Consider both the good and the bad moments of your life. Granted, I chose most often to consider the bad.

Now place those thoughts on your own life canvas. Give those thoughts a color. For simplicity purposes think of them in shades of black and white. White could be a good event, grey may be neutral, and black may be... Well, let's just say that black would be a BAD day.

Take a step back from your canvas of life; with all your tiny juxtaposed dots of white, grey, and black. What image do you see? Is the image predominantly dark? Or, maybe the image is closer to being a light grey or lighter shade of white? So what does it mean? Well, that is something we'll discover together in this book.

Worth noting from the first book is my constant fascination with a roman philosopher who lived during the second millennium. I mention how this philosopher, reached forward in time, and touched my very soul. It would be his writing, which would contribute to the passion I have today, and his writing I owe the process that I will articulate between the covers of this book.

If we're successful, this book will set the stage for enhancing the existing therapies, namely talk and medicinal. These are two very good therapies. However, I believe their effectiveness can be improved through the use of a structured process. As a person who has spent about 15 years working in the field of systems engineering, I found it quite natural to evaluate what I had done and transform those steps into what you see here today; a methodical, deliberate, three dimensional assessment of your inner self. Together, we'll use the concepts bestowed on us from an old roman Philosopher and a French Post-Impressionist painter. They will give us the basis for the tools we need to evaluate ourselves.

Thank you for choosing this book. Thank you for realizing mental wellness can come in many forms and from many sources. Mine is simply just one of those many.

Chapter 1. A Philosopher, a Painter, and a Young Boy.

Section 1: How did I get here?

I'll not likely forget the discussion I had with my wife and daughter now many months ago. I was writing my first book and working on the Preface. Not an avid reader myself, I was naive to the nuances many readers have as they approach a new read. My approach to reading is a simple one, I'll read the front and back cover of a book. I'm very fortunate that my wife and daughter are avid readers. They can plow through a book in a matter of days. Needless to say, I had a lot of learning to do when it came to book structure. I had to search on the term, just to find information on what sections make up a book exactly. I framed my first book around the result of that search.

One of those many sections was a preface, just like the one in this book. I labored hours on it, fine tuning each word, and each phrase until I was satisfied. That morning, sitting at the kitchen table pecking away at the laptops keyboard, my wife and daughter enter. My loving daughter politely asked, "So Pops, what's the book about?" I politely explained the subject matter. My wife then asked, "So how far are you into the writing?" I nicely explained, "Well, not that far. I just finished writing the preface." They both looked at me instantly. My wife saying, "Ah, Todd. You know most people who read books don't read the preface right?" My daughter never passing up an opportunity to pile on, "Yea Dad. No one reads the preface." I gave a kind smile back at both of them, clenched my fist, and said, "No. I didn't know that." I glanced down at my laptops screen seeing the fruits of my labor wilt away in front of my eyes. With that out of the way, and for all those "avid" readers who don't read the preface, I will expound on the themes of the preface in this chapter.

Up to this point, I have not spelled out the acronym, S.E.A.M. And, I won't here either, you'll just have to read on. I will say the reason for the periods in between the letters exist as a direct result of my search of the United States Patent and Trademark Office (USPTO). Believe it or not, the word "SEAM" is trademarked. I searched on S.E.A.M. and learned it was not, at least not that my searches revealed. I'm certain if the book gets any kind of publicity at all I'll find out for sure.

Anyone who has followed so far may realize this book represents only a portion of my work. This title is a complement to a series of planned writings. The first book, A Journey in the Fog of Depression: A Military Officer's Experience was the first installment and released in eBook form late September of 2013. This book represents the second installment. I have plans for the development of two additional titles that will complement the Journey series and utilize the S.E.A.M. process described here as a means for developing the books' content.

In the winter of 2009 I was diagnosed with severe depression. I was on active duty in the United States Navy, a Commander or O-5 at the time. It was only after my third time on a therapeutic plan when I truly had my "ah ha" moment. I guess you can say, "I found my passion." With the help and support of my wife of 25 plus years, and my five children, I was able to discover those experiences that contributed to my illness.

The road to my "ah ha" moment was not a pleasant one. Twice before I had contemplated suicide. Once, looking down from a fifth floor balcony on a dark night in Norfolk, Virginia and another, in my own home standing quietly in a darkened corner of the kitchen, I held in my hand multiple sleeping pills. If it wasn't for the interruption by my son, I'm not fully certain there would be a first book.

At the time, I felt alone, isolated, not understood, no place to go, in pain, and mentally exhausted. I was losing everything I had held so close to me. I isolated myself from my five children to the point they'd stop talking to each other when I entered the room. My relationship with my wife was collapsing around me. One late weekend afternoon, she sat crouched up against our bedroom wall, crying into her hands. As she paused from crying, she looked at me, standing in the hallway several feet away, "NO! NO! Don't do that!" As she screamed these words, she watched me as I reached down for my wedding band, and pulled it off my finger. I threw the ring saying, "I want this to STOP! I'm tired of this!" Despite this dramatic and despicable event, she remained and remains today by my side.

In another noteworthy moment, although admittedly not as serious as those two just mentioned, I found myself stopped behind a white SUV on a wet and stormy night. The traffic light had just changed from red to green. The white SUV did not move. Several seconds passed and the SUV still did not move. The rain pounding on the windshield, the wipers rhythmically sweeping by my eyes as I looked at this SUV. My pulse began to race, my hands began to sweat, and I felt threatened. A feeling that my very life would be in danger if I didn't act, if I didn't do something. I reached down for the gear shift, pressed down on the clutch with my left foot and placed the car in reverse. I quickly looked behind me and with my heart racing I backed up. Suddenly, the car jolts forward. I had unknowingly hit a vehicle that was just behind me. As the car settled to a stop it was as if someone had snapped their fingers to wake me from a hypnotic state. I couldn't believe what had happened.

These were just a few moments or "waypoints" I describe in my first book. These moments plus many more, contribute to what I refer to as my Journey. I use the word "my" very lightly. One person suffering from the effects of depression does not suffer in isolation. My wife, five children, friends, and co-workers all were affected in some way by my depression. I mentioned earlier, I will explore the effect and impact on my wife and five children as the topic of two additional Journey books

Section 2: The S.E.A.M.

There I was, wallowing in my desperate emotions, and nowhere to turn. I'd been in and out of therapy twice already by this time. Each time was preceded by a more devastating event. Devastating to my wife, to my family, and to myself. It was only after nearly ending my marriage I finally realized; I finally had a logical thought, "I have to get back into therapy. I have to try it yet again. If I don't get help I'll simply head back down another self-destructive path."

One of those "self-destructive" paths for me was exercising to excess or, exercising to extremes. I was working out seven or eight times a day, each time for about one hour or more. I had lost about 40lbs. My "waypoints" at the time, would have taken me on a collision course with the metaphorical rocky shoreline if I didn't change my course, and change it soon.

I convinced myself, as well as others, I was fine. Every day I put on the uniform I slipped deeper and deeper into the character of my former self. I acted the character every day. When I removed the uniform, I would slip into the darkness of the fog. A Jekyll and Hyde effect of sorts. Although, I had missed one thing, one crucial piece of my master plot to destroy my life. I neglected the effect my appearance would have on my cover. Yes, my physical appearance. I was too cheap to go out and buy new uniforms to cover up the skin that was simply acting as a bed sheet for my bones. There's only so much a person can do to hide a slowly disintegrating body. I realized I had to change up the script. I acknowledged others who might ask about my depleting appearance, "Oh, I'm fine. I'm just having some medical issues. It's not life threatening though. Thanks for asking." "Not life threatening," this couldn't have been further from the truth. The fact was I wanted to die. I even thought if I died from over exercising it wouldn't be considered a suicide. I believed this to be the perfect suicide. It would protect my family from the stigma associated with the act, while not giving the general populace the indication I was truly a coward. My death would just be a tragic and unfortunate instance in time, a final "waypoint".

There were several factors contributing to my rationale for leaving therapy. I mentioned the stigma, the negative energy, or gravitas. There was also the effect my diagnosis would have on my career as a Naval Aviator, my security clearance, and my pay.

One more factor was the inability to find value in Talk Therapy. Talk Therapy to me, provided no means to an end. It had the appearance of some perpetual process with no framework, no map, and therefore no end in sight.

I needed someone to give me a map or a plan. Maybe it was the old navigator in me, which gravitated towards waypoints and fixes. I needed to understand where I had been, where I was going, and when I would get there. The thought of a map or plan was balanced with the need for a documented process. I attribute this desire to my 15 plus years in the field of Systems Engineering. Those many years in this engineering discipline taught me the importance of frameworks, models, and analysis.

I had to understand the process or the methodology leading me to a cure. I needed the ability to visually see where I was and where I was going. This need for visual cues and process lead me to where we are today.

The tragedy of it all was, instead of seeking help, I found myself pulling away from it. During my appointments I was often met with a, "How are you today?" or "What brings you in today?" or "What would you like to talk about today?" When the therapist and I would engage in dialogue, I would often see their face appear confused by the military terms I'd use.

Another important factor in the tearing away from therapeutic help was attitude, bias, or a personal mindset. I grew up thinking therapists were folks wearing long white doctor's coats, held a clip board in their hand, spoke with a European accent, and had a long cushy couch in their office. This was completely incorrect and was simply wrong. It's not the therapist that have the couches…..It's the psychiatrist. The therapists have only the cushy chairs.

I say all of this, acknowledging the fact, I TRULY believe each person I met along the way, was fully qualified and professional. I simply wasn't connecting. I discovered over time within the acquisition world, and the same is true with many professions, there is a vernacular, a language. If you don't know the language, you are behind the curve, and often left confused and in the dark. Without a connection I knew it wouldn't go anywhere, wherever "anywhere" was. These factors just discussed, collectively, contributed to my irrational reasoning.

Considering all of what has just been written let me create a mental picture of what was happening, relative to my own experience with the therapies:

Take a scrap of paper, any size or color will do. Now fold that piece of paper in half. Run your thumb nail down the crease and tear the paper so you have two halves. Take a couple pieces of tape. Place the tape along the seam of the two pieces so that now your previously two pieces are whole again. Draw a stick figure on the left side of the seam. On the right hand side, draw a circle and another stick figure.

The stick figure on the left side represents YOU or the person seeking treatment. The stick figure on the right represents the Therapist and the circle represents the available medications to help treat depression.

This is the really fun part. Hold the piece of paper in front of you, grabbing the top corner of each half. With a slight force begin to pull in down and in the opposite direction. What happens to the seam? What happens to the two pieces of paper? The stick figure on the left? The stick figure on the right? The circle representing the medications?

With just a scrap of paper, a piece of tape, a pencil, and an ever so small amount of elbow grease, we just replicated what happened to me over, and over again. Figure 1, Illustration of the seam, provides a graphic depiction of the concept.

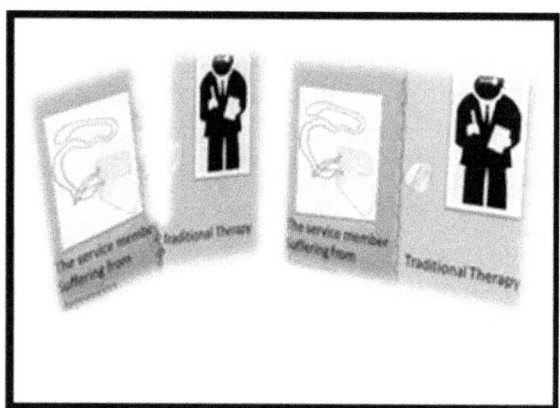

Figure 1. Illustration of the seam.

Those factors we discussed: the stigma, the pay, the effect on career, and the lack of connection with my therapist. They gave the force a magnitude vector or amperage. The force described ripped me away from those things I had at one time held so close. A force, ripping me from the help I so desperately needed. I wasn't prepared for it. I wasn't expecting to engage such a menacing foe.

Fortunately for me, I returned to therapy for yet a third time. I knew this time had to be different. This time was the only thing between me and my imminent death.

We will often refer back to this concept of a seam through the course of this book. Meaning, the virtual crease, or seam existing between the patient and current therapies. Recognizing this seam was critical in my treatment plan. Realizing what happens when it is breached, was even more critical.

In the engineering world, a seam is a design weakness, a location deserving additional attention and analysis. Just as in the building of fuel cells for aircraft. Seams are bonded and overlapped to prevent leakage and withstand the forces of a possible mishap condition.

Thanks to a few serendipitous events, I realized just how you can reinforce the seam, bind it tightly, so as to remove any chance of it being torn away again. How I got there will be the topic of future chapters and is the essence behind why I'm writing this book.

This book, along with the other companion writings, may or may not help you specifically. I only hope by reading these words, finding interest in the topic, you just might find some value, find a few nuggets of thought that just might trigger you to stop and realize help is out there. There is a way out of the fog.

Section 3: Lucius Seneca the Younger.

I happened to stumble upon this man, this man called Lucius Seneca the Younger. Lucius Seneca the Younger, pictured in the below figure, was a Roman Stoic philosopher who later in his life became an advisor to Emperor Nero. An important fact, Nero was convinced Seneca the Younger was contriving to kill him. So, Nero ordered Seneca to commit suicide.

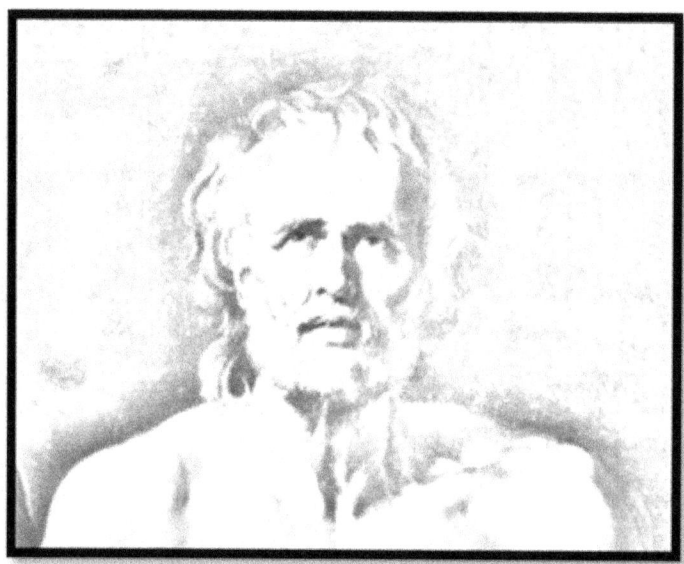

Figure 2. Lucius Annaeus Seneca the Younger.

How I came across such a man in history is quite amazing. I was deep into the fog of depression. I sat alone on our couch in the family room with my laptop as the only light in the otherwise darkened room. I was struggling with my faith. I realized the faith I had grown up with wasn't sufficient for me. I needed something that had a basis in logic. I felt as though my faith was contributing to my lies. I was living a faith which I couldn't logically comprehend. I saw the robes and the ceremony as needless pomp and circumstance. I couldn't believe there would be an almighty being requiring I bow before him (or it). Ok, required may be a strong word here.

I recently watched a segment on one of those cable shows. A priest was being interviewed by the host about the upcoming Catholic Youth festival. From what I could gather the Pope had "tweeted" that if you watch the Catholic Youth Festival on the Internet you could be saved from going to purgatory. What? Are you kidding me? Is the Almighty so powerful and wonderful that he would cause one to have to make a pit stop on the way to Heaven? Really? The younger looking priest continued to banter with the host. I couldn't help but think to myself, "Was he really believing what he was saying? A purgatory? I began to search for alternatives."

I searched through the World Wide Web and I came across a multitude of religious faiths. I read about the Protestant, the many Christian groups, the Quakers, and Pantheism. Pantheism you say? I'd be surprised if many know the word. I came across it on many of my searches. I began to focus my reading on the pantheist. I have to admit, I liked what I read. It was actually making sense to me.

Much like the Stoics of Lucius' day, the Pantheist believe everything is attributable to an all-encompassing being (you can call it God if you would like). I've also read it another way, "That the universe or nature is identical with divinity." Once I came across this passage I said to myself, "Ah, now I have found myself. The universe, nature, of course it's god like. Of course it all makes sense to me now." Ok, maybe I'm jumping the gun, but I had to admit it did make more sense.

You're wondering when I'll get to the point. I began by talking about a Roman philosopher who advised the emperor Nero and now I'm talking about religion. Well, while I searched on Pantheism I came across a quote attributed to Lucius Seneca the younger. Remember, the Stoics belief system was closely related to that of Pantheism so it was quite reasonable for me to find this quote.

What is the highway to freedom? Any vein in your body. – *Lucius Annaeus Seneca the Younger*

The quote above was so powerful to me that I read it over, and over, and over again. Those words summed up how I was felt at the time. The highway to freedom, to peace, was in death, my death. Lights out. Turn the switch off. That's all she wrote.

How easy does he make it sound? A little slice on both wrist, and done. But is that what he intended those words to mean? Was there another way to interpret these words? Did he really mean death? Death as we know it today? Did he really mean your bodily vein? The physical vein within? I'd churn on these words many times. Even today, I think about those words and reflect on their meaning, hoping I got it right. Like it or not, Lucius found a new home with me. He joined me on my journey in the fog. He'll be with me for the duration of my journey.

Can you imagine it? In an age of cell phones, electronic tablets, and the Internet, someone who likely wrote on papyrus reached out and grabbed me with his words today. I hate to give this a rosy picture though. Remember, I'm deep in the fog of my depression when I read those words. I'm shopping for religions, my marriage is crumbling all around me, and my children won't talk with me. I was not in a good place. Here are these words. Words conveying to me a sense of happiness, a sense of true freedom. I had the ability to affect change in my life. I could go back to nature, back to the universe, the divine. I'll admit these thoughts drove me deeper into the darkness of my depression. About this time, I recall standing in the darkness of the corner of our kitchen, holding a sleeping pill bottle in one hand, and a handful of the very same pills in the other. This is how a man, who lived millennia ago, affected my life today, in 2013.

We'll discuss Lucius some more in a later chapter and how I was able to draw parallelism to his quote. Lucius is actually one reason for me being here today.

Section 4: Georges-Pierre Seurat

We just discussed the influence a man, who lived in the 2nd millennium, and how his words influenced my thinking today. The next influence starts out a bit comical. Literally, it starts out with a cartoon. A cartoon character named, *Magilla Gorilla*. Allow me to explain.

Growing up in the suburbs of Chicago, I grew up with television. Television was to my generation as the Internet is to this generation, it was just as self-absorbing. Television allowed us to imagine ourselves somewhere else, it was informative, and of course entertaining to watch.

Growing up before cable meant you were limited to commercial stations. Some were the big name national networks we have today, while others were local stations. A few of these local stations were transmitted in the Ultra High Frequency (UHF) band. They offered older shows. We'd refer to them today as, the classics. One of these classics was the cartoon Magilla Gorilla; a series that originally ran in the 1960's. There's a catchy tune associated with the show as well, but I'll save you from having to read through it here and allow you to do your own surfing to find out more. Suffice it to say, "How much is that Gorilla in the window?" Sorry, I just couldn't help myself.

I have never forgotten a commercial shown on one of these local television stations. While watching this local station, one of my favorite cartoons was being broadcast. In between the cartoons segments, the local station televised an educational commercial. The commercial began with a panned out image of a painting while accompanied by an announcer who provided some voice over. The camera panned in on the picture, closer, closer, and even closer. Suddenly, the viewer began to make out distinctive dots. Tiny, individual, and colored dots. Dots so close to one another, you found it incredibly impossible that there was anyone so talented, someone who had such precision in their hands. There, on the television, was a painting. A painting made up of thousands upon thousands of colored dots. When the camera panned out the viewer could see a complete image on a canvas. The painting shown was, *Sunday Afternoon on the Island of La Grande Jatte - 1884*, Figure 3.

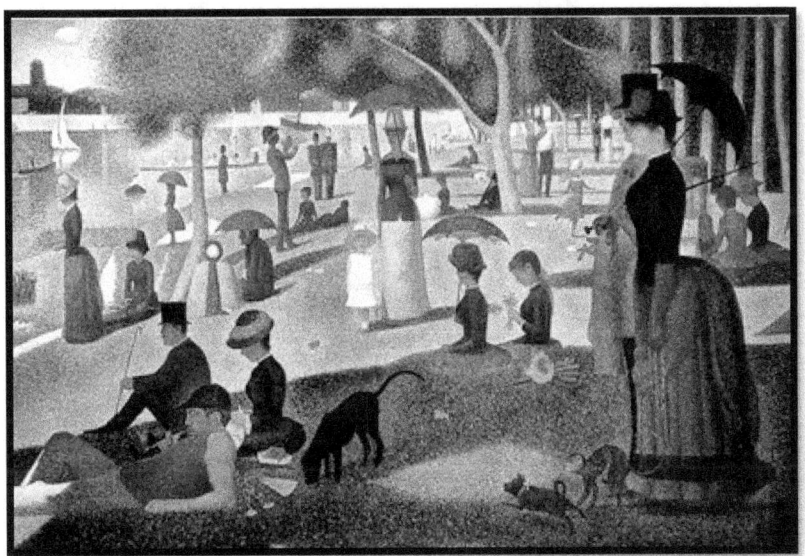

Figure 3. Sunday Afternoon on the Island of La Grande Jatte – 1884.

I thought to myself, "How cool is that!" The announcer provided more details and I heard the following words, Seurat Dots. I'll never forget those words, Seurat Dots. Maybe that's why I still recall the commercial and the genius today.

The painting displayed on the television screen was painted by the French Post-Impressionist painter, Georges-Pierre Seurat, hence the term "Seurat Dots". Seurat lived in the mid to late 1800's, a lot closer to 2013 than 4 BC was. Figure 4 labeled, *Portrait, Georges Seurat* the genius man himself.

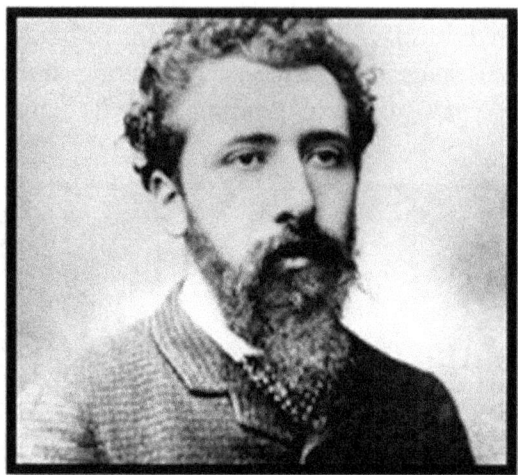

Figure 4. Portrait, Georges Seurat

I found myself affected by someone who wasn't even alive today. I'll go into much more detail with the influence our French Post-Impressionist painter had on me in a later chapter. Remember the words as I have today, "Seurat Dots."

Section 5: Parallelism.

This is the time in a fireworks display I may go, "Ohh" and "Ahh", as I watch the rockets shoot into the night sky and burst into a fiery multi colored spectacle in front of my eyes. I know, I still haven't told you what S.E.A.M. means and maybe you won't be as impressed as the fireworks finale I just described, but here goes nothing.

In earlier sections I discussed how I tore myself away from therapy, twice in fact. I also describe how my depression sent me on a search to find religion. In that search, I discovered Pantheism, a belief that nature and the universe are in fact God or the divine. While searching on the subject of Pantheism, I blindly stumbled on a saying written by a Roman Philosopher who lived around 4 BC. Then, there was the cartoon of a Gorilla. The cartoon that for some reason I couldn't get out of my head. I couldn't figure out why I kept thinking about the cartoon. Then it dawned on me, it wasn't the cartoon at all, it was the informative commercial in the middle. A commercial depicting the works of a particular French painter; Georges Seurat, and his painting of a Sunday Afternoon. Figure 5, below labeled, *The seam puzzle*, illustrates these various seemingly disparate puzzle pieces.

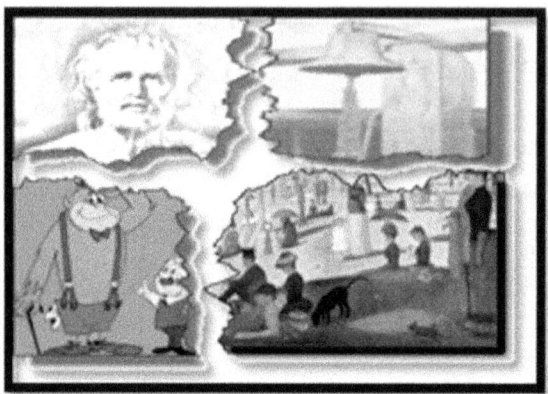

Figure 5: The seam puzzle.

I must circle back just one more time before all of this can make some sense.

I was now in therapy for the third time. I mentioned to my therapist I was having some issues. I had gone to the Flight Doc a week prior and asked to have my meds increased to 200mg. I mentioned this fact to the therapist, I told her how I was getting up at 3:00 or 4:00 AM, and sitting in our family room alone and in the darkness. Alone, lights off, and just thinking; a destructive combination for someone who has severe depression. I felt the fog of my depression slowly coming back and surrounding me, engulfing me. It was a paralyzing feeling. It was frightening. Frightening because I knew what it could mean. I'd been on this journey long enough to know the signs of the fog. I knew the waypoints. I plotted the course in my head and I knew they only led to my ultimate demise.

My Therapist mentions, "We need to find something for you to do when you're in the dark place." I thought to myself, "Yea, that sounds good. What is it?" She then said, "I would normally recommend exercise but….I wouldn't in your case." I'd lost about 40 pounds and now weighed a mere 145 pounds. I had been working out anywhere from six to eight times a day. Working out to excess was my path to self-destruction. Suicide by working out to excess… Sounded good to me at the time. I'd be the healthiest dead person around.

She looked back at me as I sat in the comfy chair, "Well, how about yoga?" She paused then said, "Well, we're just brainstorming here." Then she said, "How about reading. I have some books here that you may like." Once again my non-verbal communication skills must have been in full force that session. I mentioned at the beginning of the chapter, I was not considered an avid reader, not by a long shot. I began to feel badly about how this was going. I realized she was trying to help. The suggestions just were not clicking with me. I left the session thinking, "Wow, I don't have a life. I don't have anything that I like to do outside of work. Yoga, reading, and even working out was now off the proverbial table…. What can I do?"

I walked back to my car and I began to replay our session in my head. I thought once again about what we discussed and her suggestions. With working out now removed from the list, it left two suggestions on the table. The first was yoga. Again, a great suggestion for someone who may be Gumby or Pokey which I was neither; so I ruled out yoga. That left reading. There are avid readers and there is ME. If avid described the one extreme of the reading scale I would be the lower end of that same scale. Yes, my name would show up as NOT a reader. Maybe it's part of my personality. I never had the patience or attention span to read. I always seemed to jump to the end of a book or simply buy the Cliff Notes version.

Our children, like many, loved it if Mom or Dad would read a story to them. I'd say to one of the kids, "Why don't you go grab a book form the bookshelf and Dad will read to you." I'd either be sitting on the couch or in a wing back chair. One of the kids would make the climb up on my lap, carrying a book tucked tightly towards their chest, while I'd reach out with both hands, grab them gently under the arm, and give them the last boost they needed to climb up.

The books were often old and worn. Five children and always a dog in the house, you can imagine the wear they went through. I was normally familiar with the story since it was either read to them the night before or was read multiple times in the past to one of the now older children. Out of the blue it hit me, the sleep monster. I would begin to read, my eyes would begin to feel heavy, and heavier, and heavier until, low and behold they were shut tight. I would only be awakened by the bellow of, "MOM! DAD FELL ASLEEP, AGAIN!" So books were out as well.

My mind drifted to one particular high school English class and one very specific assignment. I remember the assignment very distinctly. We were given a creative writing assignment. For those that read the first book, you will not be surprised by the topic I chose to base my writing on. War, of course.

The evening before the assignment was due I was sitting down in my childhood home's basement bedroom thinking about a story. A number of war movies played through my head. I started to think about a story. I began to think about what parents of soldiers must have felt like state side knowing their children were in harm's way overseas. I thought about the daily routine of life in the states and how it contrasted to life in a war zone. I began scribbling my thoughts down on paper (we didn't have computers yet). I imagined a soldier standing inside one of those landing crafts. The soldier, reflecting back on what life was like in his Iowa hometown. He thought about his mother and the chores she'd be doing at that very instant in time. He thought about his father. As he had these thoughts, he began to hear the artillery rounds hitting the water on all sides of the landing craft. He could already hear the cries and screams emanating from the landing craft nearby. As they hit the water, he could hear his father back home begin to chop wood. The mullet, hitting the wood with a loud crushing sound, splintering the wood into small pieces which flung into the air.

The mother, in the kitchen frying some of her best fried chicken. Sounds of the oil sizzling around the fat of the frying chicken, popping into the air are heard. A similar popping sound grabs his attention as he hears the bullets from the enemy, perched on the cliffs zero in on their landing craft.

The story ended with their son, sitting down at the table, staring at his parents as they talked. He tries to interrupt their conversation, but cannot be heard. The sound of an approaching car interrupts the dinner conversation. The parents get up from the table and head to the front door. The returning soldier follows, looking inquisitively at what was taking place. The soldier stands behind them. The car pulls up to the front of the house. A man dressed in his Class A's opens the car door and walks over to the parents. The mother begins to sob as the father places his hands on her shoulders. The son, standing near the doorway seeing this once again tries to speak, but again he cannot be heard. The Military Officer approaches the parents and tells them that "he regrets to inform them of their son's death." The son then realizes he didn't survive the landing. He begins to feel his uniform. He looks down at his chest. He sees a hole, right over his heart while a dark red blood soaked stain surrounds the entry wound. There was more but this gives an impression of what I wrote.

The day the assignments were handed back to us I recall the very same English teacher holding up my work in front of the class. "Mr. Kruder. Did you happen to copy this from somewhere?" I was in disbelief. Disbelief that my English teacher was accusing me of plagiarism. Even more disbelief that he was holding up MY paper. I swallowed hard and said, "No sir. It is my own work." He brought the paper back down to his side, "Well, it's very good. Of course there's a number of grammar and spelling errors. If it were not for those I would have given you a higher grade."

I'm about half way home now and I continue to consider those days in high school. I asked myself, "What about writing?" I have to admit, I had my doubts. I failed the fourth quarter of my senior year English class, squeaking by with a "D" overall. I also had to take the lowest level of English in college. I hope this confession does not deter you from reading on or reading another one of my books.

In the first book of this series I described in detail the serendipitous events that unfolded leading up to my decision to begin writing. My high school experience described here was simply the foundation for the motivation. It was that very weekend I found myself on the elliptical, watching the Sunday Morning news program at nine o'clock in the morning. The Sunday news program aired a self-publishing segment. I'd never heard of self-publishing up until this point in time.

Watching the news segment on self-publishing was the last of the signs I needed to make a decision. I thought to myself, "I had to do something. Why not writing?" I showered, went back down to the same couch I sat on all those times before, and instead of sitting in the dark, I grabbed my laptop, opened up a blank word document and simply began to type, and type, and type. After about two to three months later I had successfully compiled over 250 pages of material and a heck of a lot of grammar and spelling errors.

In between all this activity, I began to see a pattern in my writing. I started to realize I was falling back on a process oriented mind set. I spent the past 15 years working in the Systems Engineering world, process was something I understood well. One day, I opened up another blank word document, and I began to type, and type, and type. You'll never guess what came out if that effort. Yes, this book.

I found myself jotting down the steps I used when I wrote about a unique waypoint. I realized the seam that I previously described in much more detail. In between writing the two books, I also realized the connection between Lucius and Seurat.

Though they never met in real life, I felt as if the two men were in the room with me, as I pecked away at the keyboard. They were there, coaching me along, highlighting the connections between these two seemingly disparate human beings and their works of genius.

I realized those very waypoints, which described my life experiences, could resemble a dot; a dot in time, and a dot on a canvas of life. Georges Seurat was standing there, looking over my shoulder as I typed away. Seurat was whispering the words, "They are like my painted dots. They are Seurat Dots." The waypoints I was in the processing of describing were in fact, very much like those dots Seurat painted on his canvas. Those moments, just like his dots, had color, had meaning, and they had depth. I realized, at that very moment, an experience doesn't have to be just a waypoint. IT CAN BE a dot. Something I now refer to as a, "Seurat Emotional Dot."

Now it was Lucius' turn. I had a thought, "Dots with depth, color, hmmm. Maybe there was a way to characterize an event in more than one dimension." Seurat's painting technique gave a perspective of a scene, but only in one dimension. I always viewed experiences as having multiple dimensions. It became obvious to me at the time my experiences had both range and depth. Range was simply my way of thinking about time. Our experiences exist in the time domain. Depth to me indicated a thickness or diameter.

I pulled out some graph paper we happen to have nearby. I began to sketch what my brain was rapidly trying to process. I started with a circle. I add a length. I tilted the pencil on its side and shaded in some color. I looked down at the graph paper. There it was! A mere foots length away from my face. This is what Lucius and Georges Seurat were trying to tell me all along. It was starring right at me. "Oh Lucius. Oh Georges Seurat. You magnificent bastards!"

Lucius leaned over the side of the couch, pulling back his white tunic, "It's my vein. The highway to freedom." YES!!! The vein from Lucius' saying! These two geniuses, together, helped me describe what for so many years I could not understand. I looked down at the graph paper, my mind began to reel with excitement, I quickly sketched more and more; the lead from my pencil leaving small fragments on the paper from the pressure I placed on the pencil tip.

I called this epiphany a Lucius Emotional Vein. I could see the vein of my experiences now as clear as I could see the bulging blueish vein in my forearm. All derived from a simple Seurat Experience Dot.

I didn't stop there. There was still lead on the tip of my pencil. I began to graph more thoughts, more experiences, and more waypoints. Another revelation revealed itself to me that very same day, "Maybe I could develop a means to create a model of an experience. I could give it range, depth, and even color."

I started to methodically write down the various aspects of my experiences or waypoints. I discovered common elements, themes, or influences. I started to categorize them into common bins of thought. I saw a pattern develop, a frequency of use. I continued to document information from my waypoints. I began to build a process model. A model, which takes a set of unique experiences and displays them in a three-dimensional form.

I thought to myself, if I could make something like an emotion appear to be real to a person, maybe, just maybe, the person would stay on their therapeutic plan. If I could use this method to enhance the talk therapy session, maybe, just maybe they would stay with the therapy and not tear themselves away from the seam as I had done.

Just then, as if both Lucius and Seurat were speaking in unison, "It's the S.E.A.M." That's it. The Seurat Experience Analysis Model.

Some twenty plus pages later you now have it. The reason for the title, the reason for this book. How a Roman Philosopher born in the second millennium and a French Post-Impressionist painter helped me to understand the meaning behind my depression. They gave me the idea of a process, a process that could not only help me, but others as well.

Now you know the acronym and its meaning. This will be the only place and time in the book that I will spell out the acronym. You will not see it again in further chapters. Not because I don't like it or I feel it doesn't matter. No, it's because I don't want you to think of this process as just another acronym. This process is all about positively influencing the outcome of depression. It's not about a cool acronym. I have devoted myself to improving the Behavioral Health of our service members, veterans, and their families. I want the intent of this manuscript to be focused on the process and the result, NOT the acronym.

Chapter 2. The Model.

This chapter will begin our outline of the process steps. These are the very same steps I had taken within my own therapy. It was through these very steps I began to understand the complexity of an experience. It was through these steps I learned that a single moment or a compilation of moments, can linger in the far reaches of your mind; waiting for the right moment to make a reappearance, then casting you back into the fog.

I will use the very same steps in the following pages to develop the next two books in the Journey series. The third book in the series will describe my wife's experiences living with depression. The forth, and final book, will describe the impacts of depression on my five children. Each book will be based on the findings resulting from the process described here.

This is a good time to remind you of my OFFICIAL caveat. What follows IS NOT a cure for depression. This IS NOT meant in any way to replace the therapy prescribed by your professional practitioner. This is simply a tool, a method, a method that assisted me in understanding the causes of my depression. This method CANNOT stand on its own. The benefits can ONLY be realized with the help of a medical professional.

If you find value in this process, I am pleased. If you do not, please continue to search for the therapeutic method that will work for you. Above ALL, please continue on your journey and stay in your therapy.

Section 1: Setting up the environment.

I'm drawn to the memory of the film, *Karate Kid* (1984). I'm remembering the "kid" played by Ralph Macchio. He desired to be the best at karate as he could be. He found a teacher, played by the late Noriyuki "Pat" Morita. I recall the scene where Ralph Macchio is being told by Noriyuki "Pat" Morita to go wax his car, "wax on, wax off", as Noriyuki "Pat" Morita makes a circular motion with his hands. The kid's expression was one of disappointment. He wanted to start breaking boards and throwing his feet up in the air. The whole point was the teacher knew in order to be good, you must be disciplined in your approach. You just don't start breaking boards because you wear a karate gi and a colorful belt.

Much like in the movie, we will need to "wax on, wax off", only for us, it will be "breathe in, breathe out." We must discipline ourselves to relax. Our discipline will be found in our rhythmic breathing. We must also focus on the environment around us. In order to relax, the setting must be suitable. Don't believe for a second that you can relax while texting or while watching television. Ok, these things might be considered fun, but they won't get you where you need to be mentally. Therefore, consider your surroundings very carefully.

Find a room, free from distraction of all kinds. Once you find a spot, start to practice rhythmic breathing. "Practice" you say? Yes! Practice what you've been doing all your life. Consider this, the average human probably takes about 16 breaths per minute (the average person), on average we take in good ole oxygen about 960 times in just one hour or, 23,040 a day. That's a lot of breathing. Now take that number and multiply it by a year, you'd get 8,409,600 per year. Say the average person lives until they are 80 years old. That means the average person takes in 672,768,000 breaths. Now, that's a lot of breaths. I'd ask you, "How many of those breaths you just took do you remember?" Instead of breathing being simply mechanical, I suggest you think about your breaths, allowing your mind to focus. Get rid of all the clutter filling your heads every day. There's enough distractions out there. Take a few moments and think about the breaths you take, think about this moment.

Once you've found a place to call your own and you've practiced the breathing we can move on to the next step. I know, you want to get to the meat of this, as do I. Remember, "wax on, wax off." "Breathe in, breathe out."

Section 2: Getting started.

Now that we learned how to clear our minds and relax we are ready to take the first step toward finding our way out of the fog. You'll need a few things before we begin. Just like a plumber or an electrician needs their tools, we'll need our own as well. I'd recommend the following: a sharpened pencil (Either with a good eraser or a separate one. You'll be making mistakes, and that's ok), about 10 sheets of graph paper (Plain paper can work as well, although graphing paper helps for the later steps when we have to sketch), something to write on (a clip board works great), a ruler (if you like straight lines), something to make a few various sized circles with (I used a dime, nickel, and quarter), and your now clear mind.

Once we have our tools, make sure you have a few hours free. There's nothing worse than getting started and continually having stop and start again. You also do not want to feel rushed. I can't think of anything more important than your mental health and wellbeing. So why don't you make it your priority as well.

Now you have the tools, the time allotted, and the knowledge of how to clear your mind we just need to go to that place where you practiced the rhythmic breathing. Once there, put the tools down to the side, we're not quite ready yet to begin. You know what's coming next? Yep, start breathing. Do this for a few minutes until you're calm, relaxed, and at peace in your mind. Once you're there we're ready for the next step. There's a saying in the Navy when the ship is about to set sail, "Cast off the lines and prepare to make way."

Step 1. Generate your experience list.

We're now ready for the first real step in our process. The purpose of this step is to generate a list. Yes, a simple list. The list will be of those experiences you feel are important. "How do I know if they're important or not?" Good question. The safest answer is, "I don't. They're your experiences."

I offer this up for consideration. As you are now relaxed and your mind is clear. What thoughts went through your head a second ago when you read the word experiences? I know you have some, we all do. Think about it. What experiences are in your head right now, at this very moment? Don't hesitate, write them down on one of those blank pieces of paper. This is the easiest method and is exactly what I did. As an example I have included my own list as Figures 6a and 6b, *My experiences list* on the follow two page.

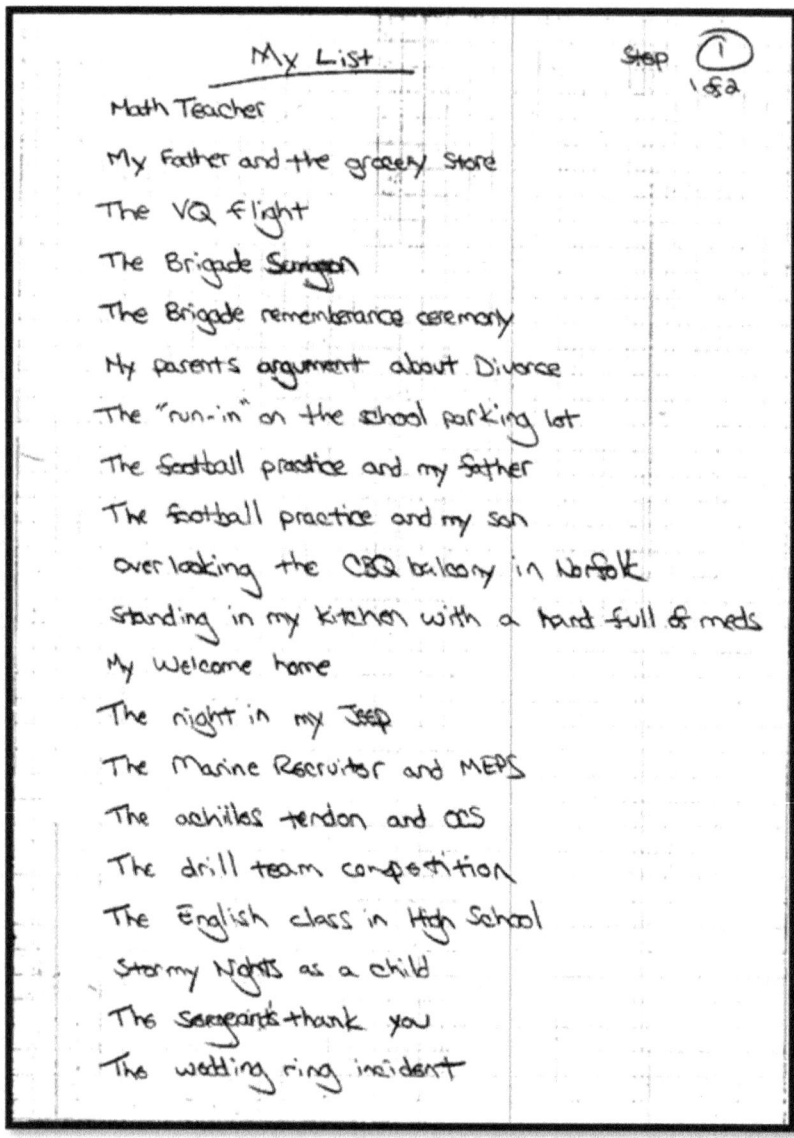

Figure 6a. My experience list.

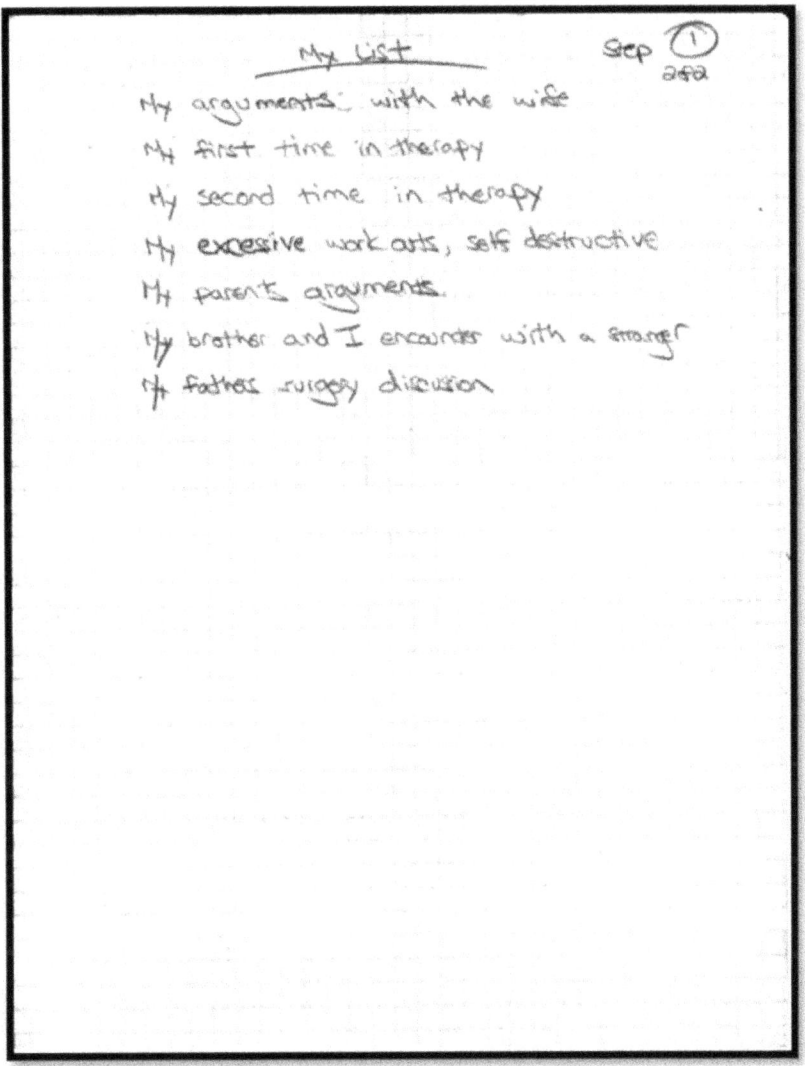

Figure 6b. My experience list.

The second method I will offer up is to consider moments in your life that had some sort of "action" either verbal or physical: a car crash, a shouting match with your spouse. Now consider these moments. Did they have an outcome associated with them? Do you remember the outcome? Write those moments down. Don't be concerned about the order just yet. We're just trying to make a good list of our experiences.

Step 2. Create a chronological experience list.

This is an important step since, we'll often refer back to the resulting timeline.

Now that you've made your list, we're going to put those experiences in chronological order. I like earliest to latest myself, but as we established earlier, "It's your list." I just offer up suggestions and examples. This is IMPORTANT, once you have transcribed your experience list chronological order, number each one sequentially. Doing so provides a shorthand reference back to the experience.

Lots of times it's difficult to remember exact dates. Exact dates aren't necessary. If you're struggling, try thinking about another event which occurred relative to the one you wrote down. Maybe your experience was near a wedding of a relative's or a graduation event. The relative timeframe is good enough right now. Remember, that's why we brought an eraser along.

Once again, this step simply results in a timeline. The next two pages present examples of my chronological list referenced as Figures 7a and 7b, *My chronological experiences.* They also demonstrate some of the juggling you might have to do at this point. Can you see my eraser marks? They're there, trust me.

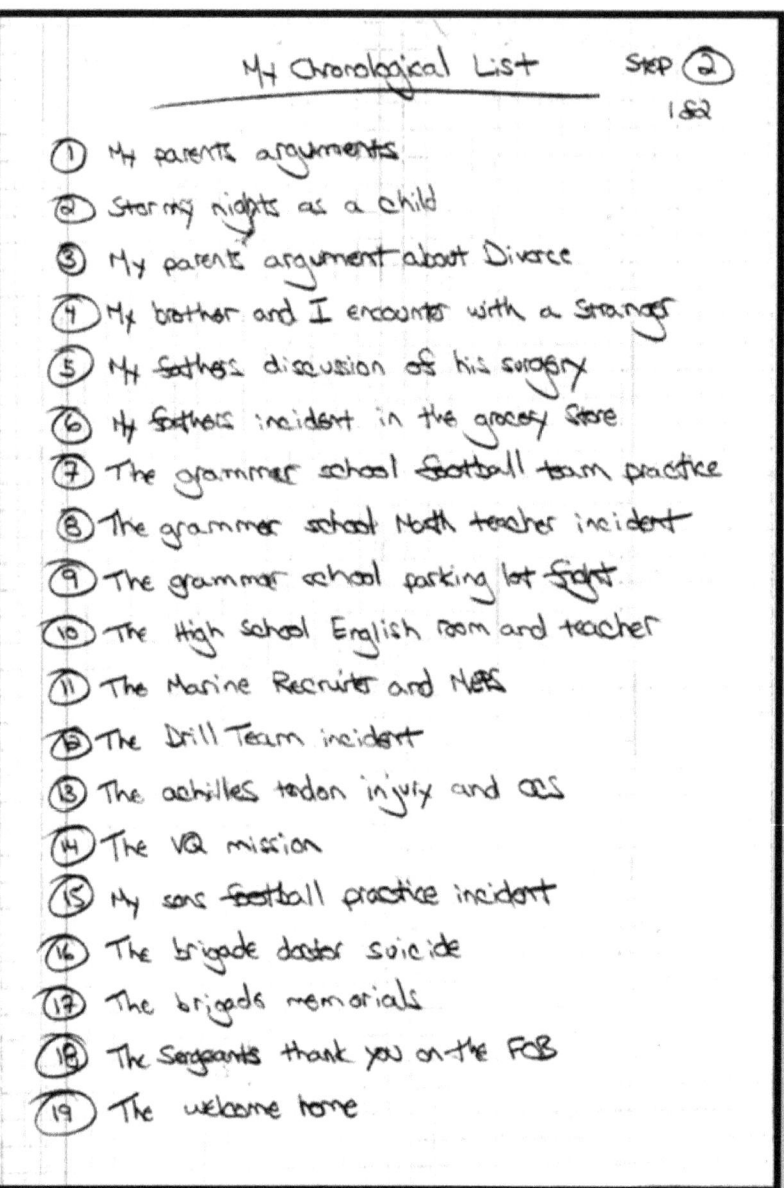

Figure 7a. My chronological experience list.

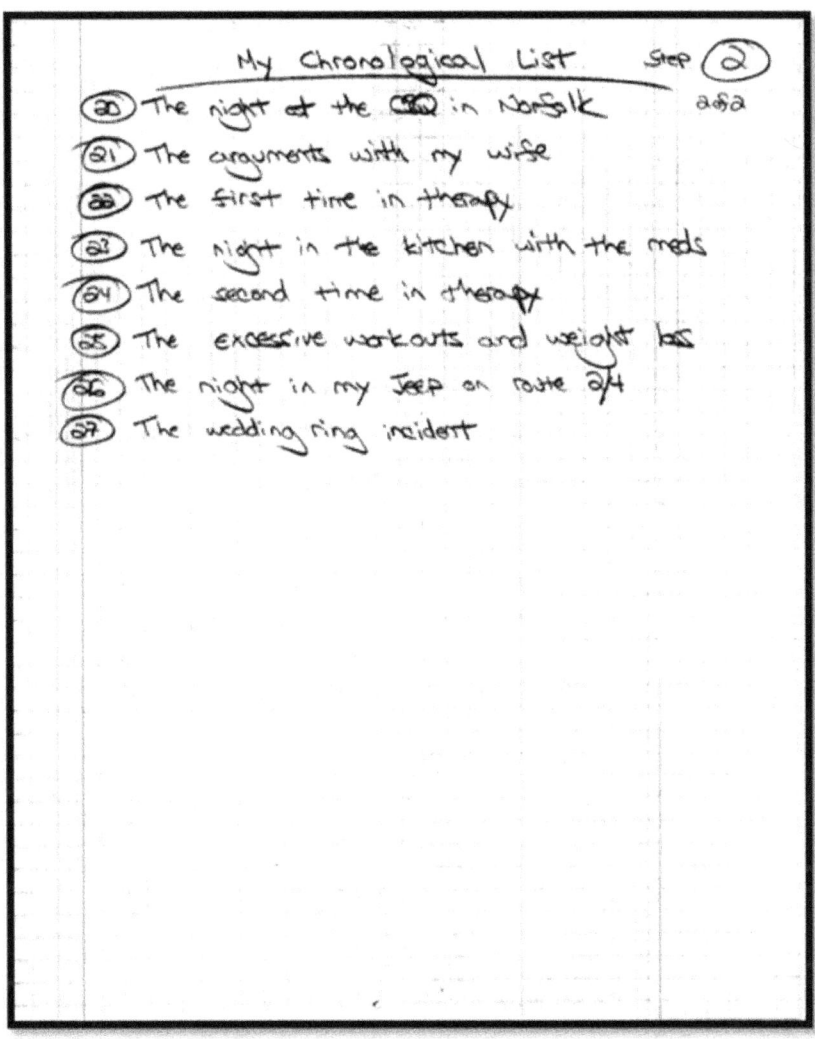

Figure 7b. My chronological experience list.

Section 3: Experience decomposition development.

The steps that follow will allow you to analyze your experiences from multiple perspectives. Before we can move onto Step 3 in our process we'll need to discuss a few topics and agree to some ground rules.

If you think about it, an experience or an event is made up of various influences. Most everything around us is an influence. We're influenced by radio, television, music, poetry, paintings, books (like this one I hope), the weather, the location or setting, the people, and even time. Yes time.

The duration or exposure during the event has an impact. I recall as a child going to the pool and having a blast playing in the water only to find out several hours later I turned into a crispy critter. Not a good thing might I add. The point here is, exposure or time matters. Duration has an effect on the outcome.

This brings us to the next important point before we move on to the third step. Outcomes. I'd like to think my life is not much different from anyone else's. I get up, put my pants on one leg at a time, just like everyone else. Consider for a moment, "a moment".

What is a moment really other than the collection of influences concentrated in the time domain. How can we distinguish a moment of time from any other? I like to think of life experiences as a collection of moments defined by a collection of influences. A collection of moments involving action(s) and a result(s) or outcome(s).

We have now established an initial train of thought. Let's discuss the various types of influences. This is going to be very important to understand hence the lengthy dissertation devoted to this step.

We'll need to agree on some basic principles and what we'll call our Influence Hierarchy. The influences I have identified here are developed based on my own perspective, your perspective may vary. Therefore, the influences categories you choose may vary as well.

I will begin by developing an Influence Hierarchy. Think of the Influence Hierarchy as a wedding cake. The hierarchy will gradually expand beneath the tier above it, just like the wedding cake. I've developed our top tier Influence Hierarchy in Figure 8 below labeled, *Top tier influence categories.*

- Top Tier Influence Categories
  - Duration
  - Emotion(s)
  - Environment
  - Personality

Figure 8. Top tiered influence categories.

The first of our four top tiered influences will be duration. Just like the sunburn story I mentioned previously, think of duration in terms of exposure time. As the earth rotates about its axis around the sun, we get closer, and we get further away through the course of day. If a person were to sun bath just after high noon on a mid-eastern summer afternoon. The person will require less time to burn than say someone who chooses a much earlier or later time in the same day. How long an experience lasts for is important.

My sense is it would be perfectly fine to say, "My experience never stopped. It haunts me today." That's ok. We'll deal with it just fine.

The second category in our hierarchy is emotion(s). Notice I placed the "s" in brackets. I suspect we all feel multiple emotions within any given moment. I only hope you're not feeling the emotion associated with boredom at this very moment. If so, I beg your forgiveness. On the following page I've listed some common emotions in Figure 9, labeled *A common emotions list.*

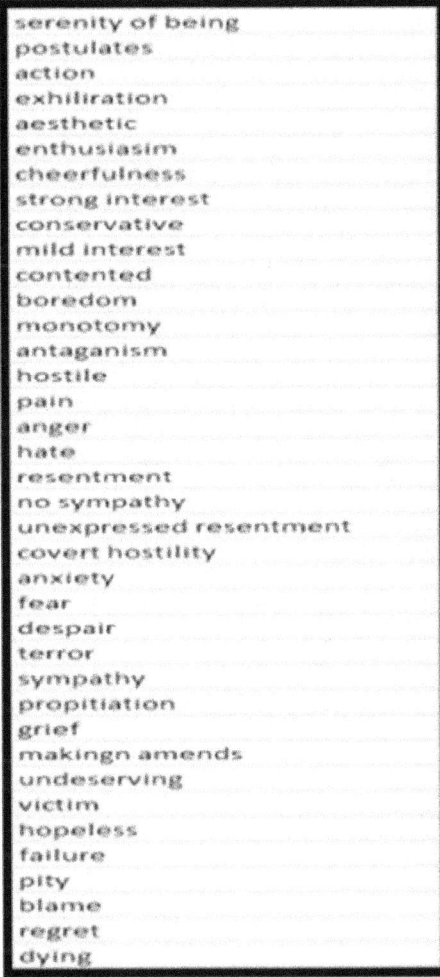

Figure 9. A common emotions list.

Do you notice something about the ordering of the emotions listed in Figure 9? The emotions are more severe as you proceed from the top to the bottom of the list.

Before anyone tells me there is an emotion missing, please don't. There are likely emotions out there not on this list. Once again, this is just a convenient list to start from, there's nothing wrong with generating your own, in fact, I encourage you to do so.

The third influence category is environment. This category is likely to be the most debated of the four listed in Figure 8. Environment can mean something different to each of us. Based on the development of my waypoints in the first book I decided to split environment influence into sub categories. Figure's 10a and 10b labeled, *Environment Influence Categories.*

- **Environment Influences**
  - **Location**
    - Rural
    - City
    - Suburban
    - Wooded
    - Desert
    - Mountainous
    - Water
      - Familiar
        - Confined / Small and enclosed space
        - Moderately Confined / Typical Classroom sized space
        - UN-Confined / Open space
      - Unfamiliar
        - Confined / Small and enclosed space
        - Moderately Confined / Typical Classroom sized space
        - UN-Confined / Open space
      - Environmental Climate Conditions
        - Temperature
          - Severe Heat (greater than 102 degrees F)
          - Hot (85-101 degrees F)
          - Mild (69 -84 degrees F)
          - Cool (52-68 degrees F)
          - Cold (32-51 degrees F)
          - Sever Cold (less than 32 degrees F)
        - Weather Conditions
          - Clear
          - Overcast
          - Light Rain
          - Heavy Rain
          - Light Snow
          - Heavy Snow
          - Sleet
          - Ice
          - Thunder Storm
          - Tropical Storm
          - Hurricane
          - Tornado

Figure 10a. Environment Influence Categories (Location)

- Environment Influence
  - People
    - Familiar
      - Family
        - Immediate
          - Father – Include Step-Father
          - Mother – Include Step-Mother
          - Brother – Include Step-Brother
          - Sister – Include Step-Sister
          - Spouse
            - Husband – Include Ex-Husband
            - Wife – Include Ex-Wife
          - Children / Grand Children
            - Son(s)
            - Daughter(s)
      - Friends
        - Known to you less than 1 year
        - Known to you for more than 1 – 5 years
        - Known to you for more than 6 or more years
      - Peers / Coworkers / Students
      - Superiors
      - Subordinates
    - Un-Familiar
      - By Standers
        - Between 1-4
        - Between 5-10
        - Between 11-20
        - Between 21-50
        - More than 51
      - First Responders / EMS

Figure 10b. Environment Influence Categories (People)

The last of the four categories used in our process is personality. There may be some contention for this category as well, I realize that. There is a lot of scientific data out there on personality characteristics. There are also a plethora of personality test as well, some more extensive than others. I do not intend to contradict or dismiss those studies and test. For my purposes, I found the simple approach works just fine. Figure 11 below labeled, Personality traits (Me) provides a sense of what I mean.

- Personality Traits
  - Shy / Reserved / Introvert
  - Mild Mannered
  - Outgoing / Extrovert

Figure 11. Personality traits (Me).

Step 3. Experience decomposition overview.

In this step we'll use everything we've just discussed. I recommend printing out the previous Figures 9, 10a, 10b, and 11. We'll refer to them frequently. The following four pages include my own experience decomposition labeled as Figures 12a through 12d, *My experience decomposition*. Once again they are provided as a reference and as an example.

This is a good time to grab some more blank sheets of paper, we'll need it. On a fresh sheet of paper, and with your own Chronological Experience List by your side, write down just the number one. Remember, there's no need to re-write the experience, we now have a key that allows us to ref back the number to the experience and vice versa. Now, whenever you see the number "one" listed, you will know two things:

1. What the experience was called.
2. A relative timeline of when that experience occurred.

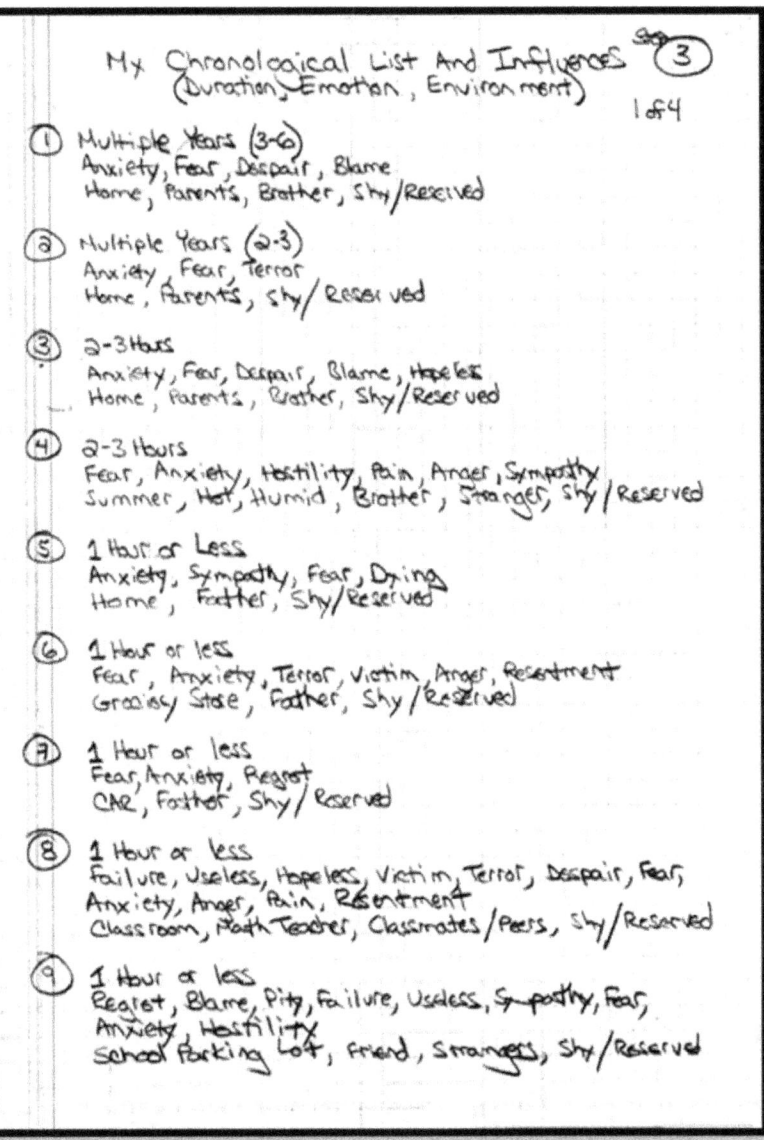

Figure 12a. My experience decomposition.

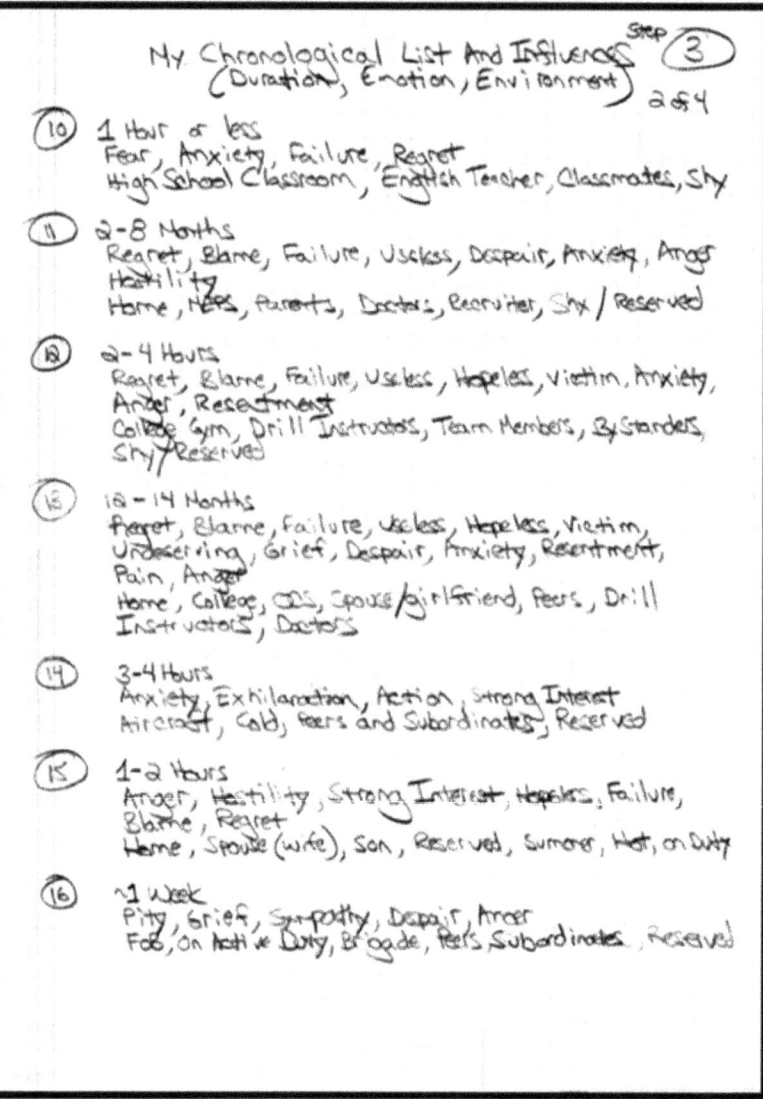

Figure 12b. My experience decomposition.

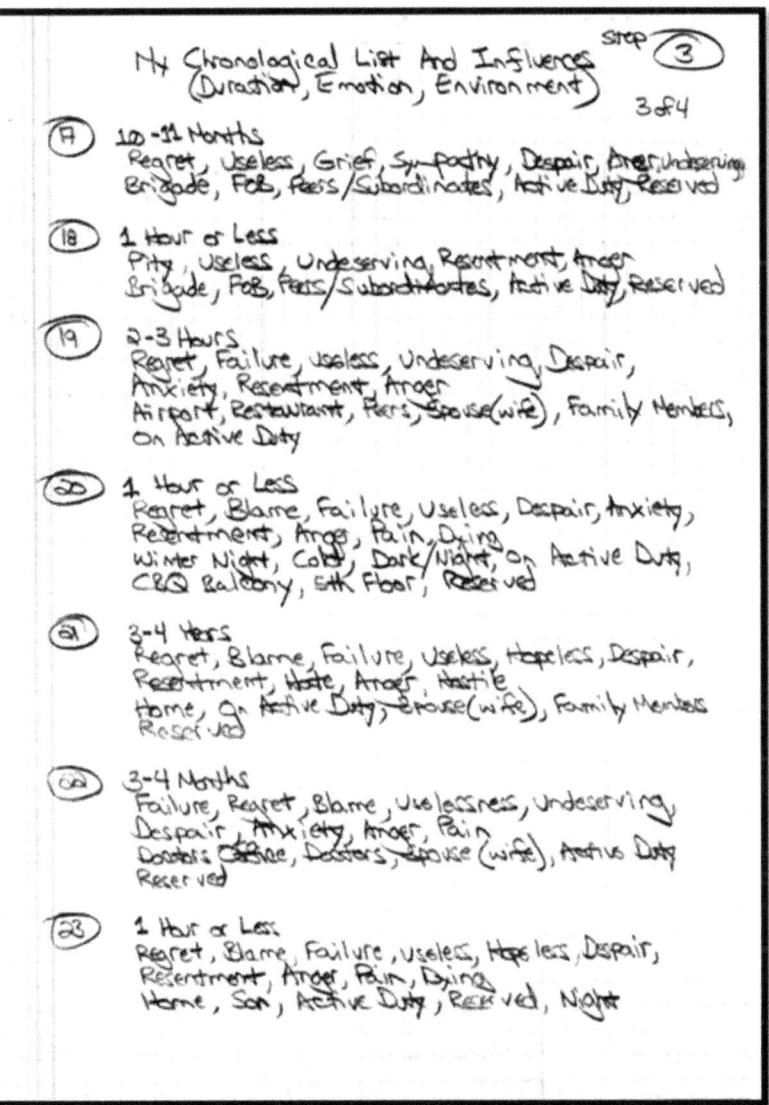

Figure 12c. My experience decomposition.

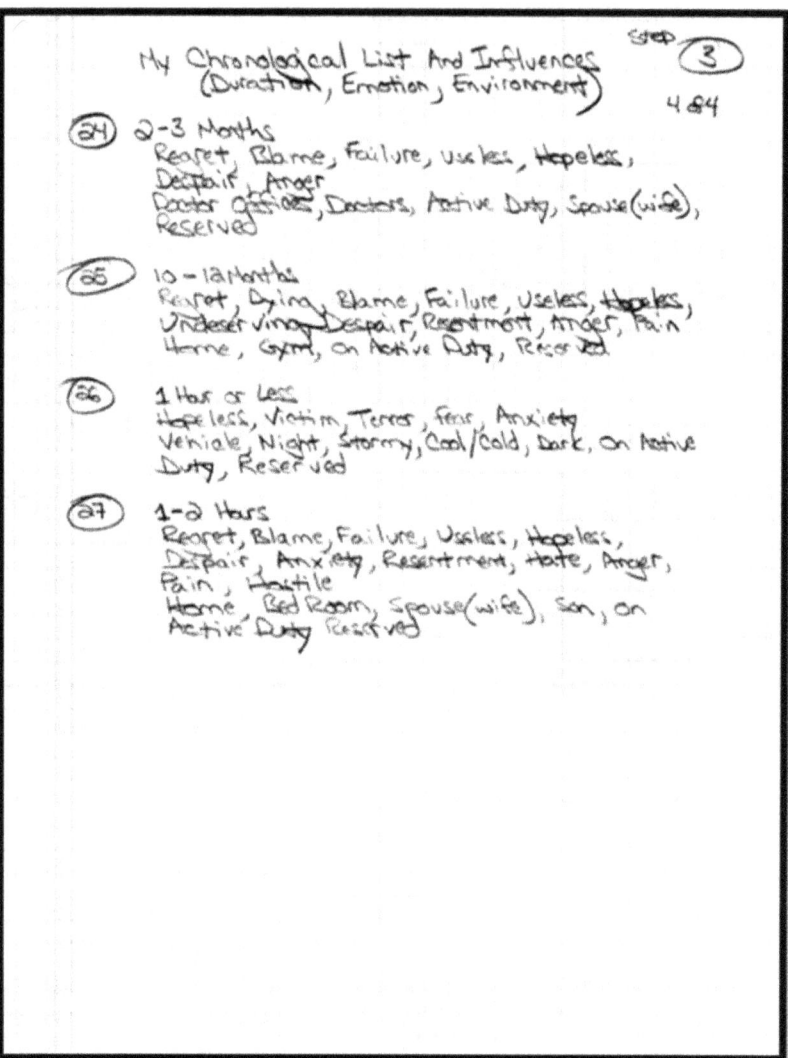

Figure 12d. My experience decomposition.

Step 3.A. Duration decomposition.

We'll start with the first of the four top tier influence areas, duration. We've got a pretty good idea based on our list when this event or experience occurred. Now, try to recall how long it lasted. Was it less than an hour? Was it two or three hours? Was it mere seconds? Or, did it occur over years? Maybe it is still going on today. Once you have a pretty good sense of the duration go ahead and make note if it below the experience. You may want to develop your own shorthand and or definitions for time. For example stick with fractions of weeks, months, years, etc. I found it useful to use terms such as; One hour or less, 2-3 hours, and Multiple years. When my experience feel across multiple years I also placed the approximate number of years in parentheses, just as a memory jogger.

Step 3.B. Emotion decomposition.

Now move onto the next category on our tiered *Influence Hierarchy*, emotion(s). Of all the influence areas we discuss I find this one to be the most compelling. Once again I highly recommend printing out the emotion list in Figure 9. Recall we discussed ho this list was ordered. The most severe emotion is listed on the bottom of the table while the least severe is listed at the top. This is important.

It's good to remind yourself of the first experience listed on our nearly clean sheet of paper. Consider each emotion listed in Figure 8. Consistency is important here. Always begin looking at the table the same way. Either start at the bottom, or start at the top. When you come across an emotion that fits your experience write it down. ITS VERY IMPORTANT TO LOOK AT THE EMOTION LIST IN FIGURE 8 THE SAME WAY FOR EACH EXPERIENCE. Doing so will make the analysis portion much easier. Here's an example what you DO NOT want to do: If I were to evaluate my first experience using Figure 8 starting at the top and work down. My emotions would likely begin with a less severe emotion and end with a more severe one. When I move onto the next experience, and this time I start at the bottom of the list in Figure 8, my emotions list will begin severe and become less severe as I proceed on. Being consistent will help significantly as we proceed on.

You'll notice in my sketches there were multiple emotions normally associated with each experience. I suspect this will likely be the case for you as well. There's no limit, write as many as you feel apply.

We now should have a piece of paper with the first of our experiences listed (one), the duration identified (remember your time annotation), and a list of applicable emotions (going from more severe to less or vice versa.).

Step 3.C. Environment (Location and People) decomposition.

We're now ready to move on and consider what environment influences may have played a part in our experiences. Let's refer back to Figures 10a and 10b for a brief moment. Environment is decomposed into two primary sub categories, location and people. I structured the factor in outline form for ease of use. For example, Figure 10a starts with Location and is decomposed further down to specific elements i.e. temperature and weather characteristics.

Once again, consider the first experience you wrote down. Try and recall the specifics of the location to the best of your ability. Did your experience occur on a rural roadway? A farm? A forested area secluded from anyone? Maybe your experience occurred on a busy street located in a downtown area of a city? Maybe it was a market place?

As we decompose the environment influences consider the familiarity of the setting. Was it familiar to you? Was it unfamiliar to you? Familiar may be relative to all of us. If you're not certain I would opt for Unfamiliar.

Further consider the environment in terms of how confined (constrained) or unconfined (unconstrained) it appeared to be. When I think of constrained I think of a car, truck, or closet. Unconstrained to me is, open to the air and the surroundings; the middle of a field or a road. The in between both of these may be a classroom, bedroom, office, etc.

Within your experience consider the true environmental influence of nature. Were you in a desert where it was extremely sunny and hot? Were you in the mountains surrounded by snow? Was it raining heavily? Was it stormy (lightening and thundering) around you? Was it foggy? If in doubt, just take a look at our initial list for a reminder of an influence consideration. You can write anything you want that best describes the environment for you. Remember, it is your experience, not mine. Just remember to be consistent across your experiences.

We'll now examine the people sub-category of environment, found in Figure 10b. This sub-category is decomposed into several sub-categories. I think we'll all agree, people play a significant part in our daily lives. They come and go through our lives, many unnoticed, many known, many we'd like to get to know better.

Look back at Figure 10b and ask yourself, "Did you know the people in the experience? Were there people you didn't know? Were there bystanders?" For those people that were familiar, were they family or friends? For those you didn't know; how many were there?

Step 3.D. The "Me" Influence decomposition.

We are now on the last of the four influence categories, personality. Take another look at Figure 11. Consider which of the traits fits YOU the best. Now look back at the experience you are evaluating. Once you feel comfortable with the choices go ahead and write it down. Remember, I call this the "Me" influence. This category is intended to provide a sense of your contribution to the experience.

Section 3 Summary.

We've now fully evaluated a single experience within the context of our four influence categories. You will need to repeat our experience analysis for each experience on your chronological experience list.

Once you've done a few it becomes very easy. The toughest part is to be consistent with how you order and annotate the influences. We'll be using this information almost exclusively in the upcoming section, *Experience decomposition analysis.*

If at any time you feel frustrated with the process, simply stop and take a break. Take a few deep breaths and try again. Remember, this is for you. This is your experience. This is your life. It's worth some reflection, trust me.

Section 4: Self-Analysis Matrix Development.

This is a good time to assess where we are on our journey of self-reflection. In Step 1 we developed a list of experiences after we found a nice quite place and practiced some relaxation breathing. In Step 2 we ordered our experience list chronologically. In Step 3 we developed an Influence Hierarchy, some associated key words, and most importantly, we decomposed each experience from step 2 utilizing that very same hierarchy, being careful to be consistent throughout.

This section, as the title suggest, is dedicated to analyzing the data we just collected. We will in essence "pivot" the data. Instead of now looking at an experience by itself and the contributing influences, we will look at each influence and the associated experience. This method will prove very telling and likely will result in some great talk therapy sessions, I'm certain.

..

Step 4. Influences vs. Experiences Correlation Matrix development.

Now that we have all this information in one location about our experiences, how about we start to organize the information. The intent will be to organize the information in such a way that we'll be able to reason on what we have, draw some conclusions, and possibly make some connections.

I've found the simplest way for me was to create a series of matrix sketches. The matrix format allowed me to view data in various aspects, from various angles; horizontally as well as vertically.

The seven pages that follow contain Figures 13a through 13g labeled *My example influence matrix*). They're provided as a reference. Your influence matrix will look different based on how you assessed the contributing influences

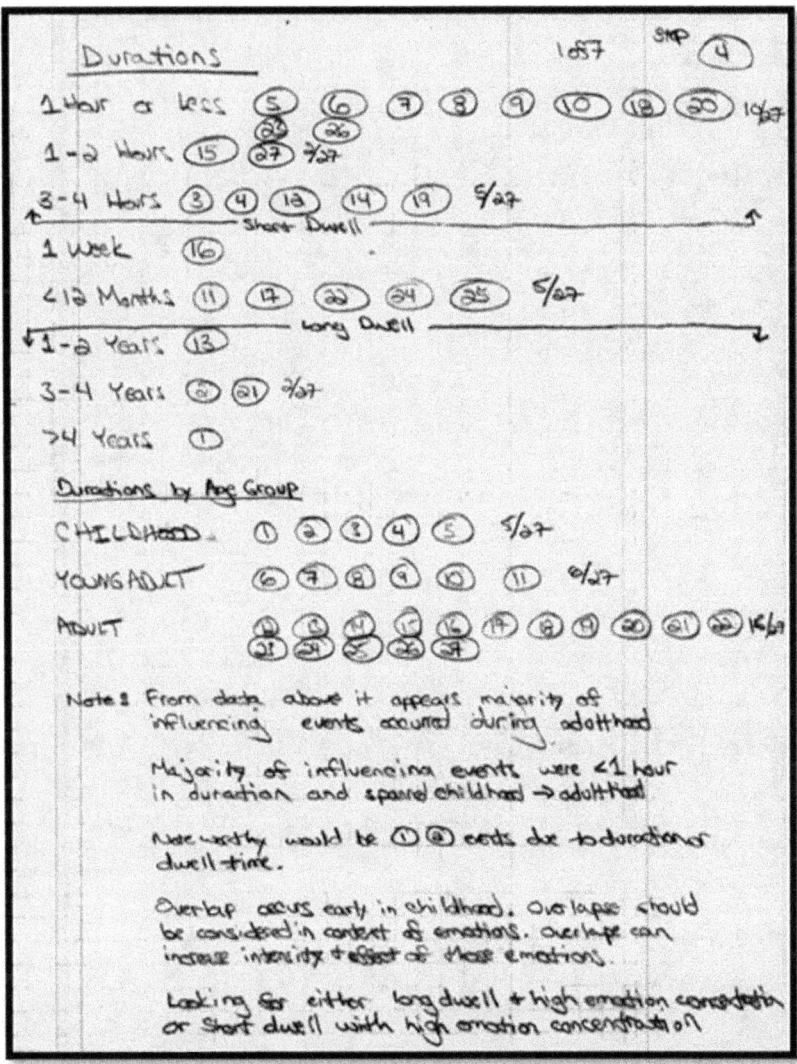

Figure 13a. My example influence matrix.

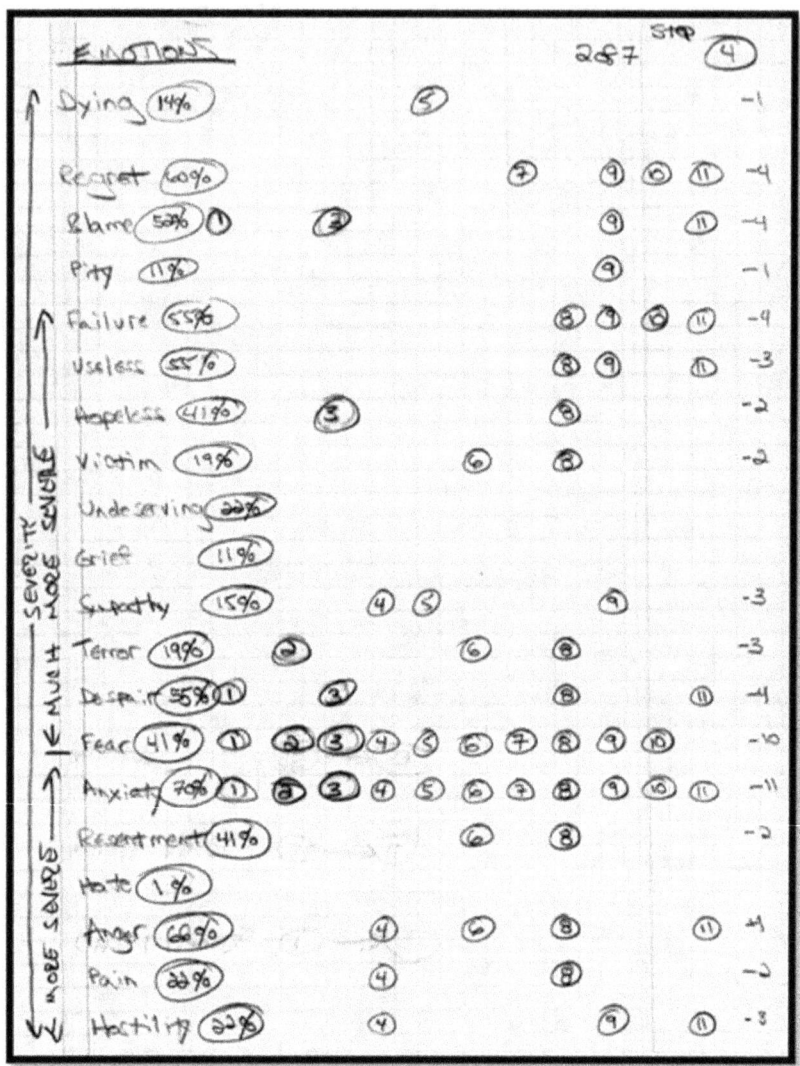

Figure 13b. My example influence matrix.

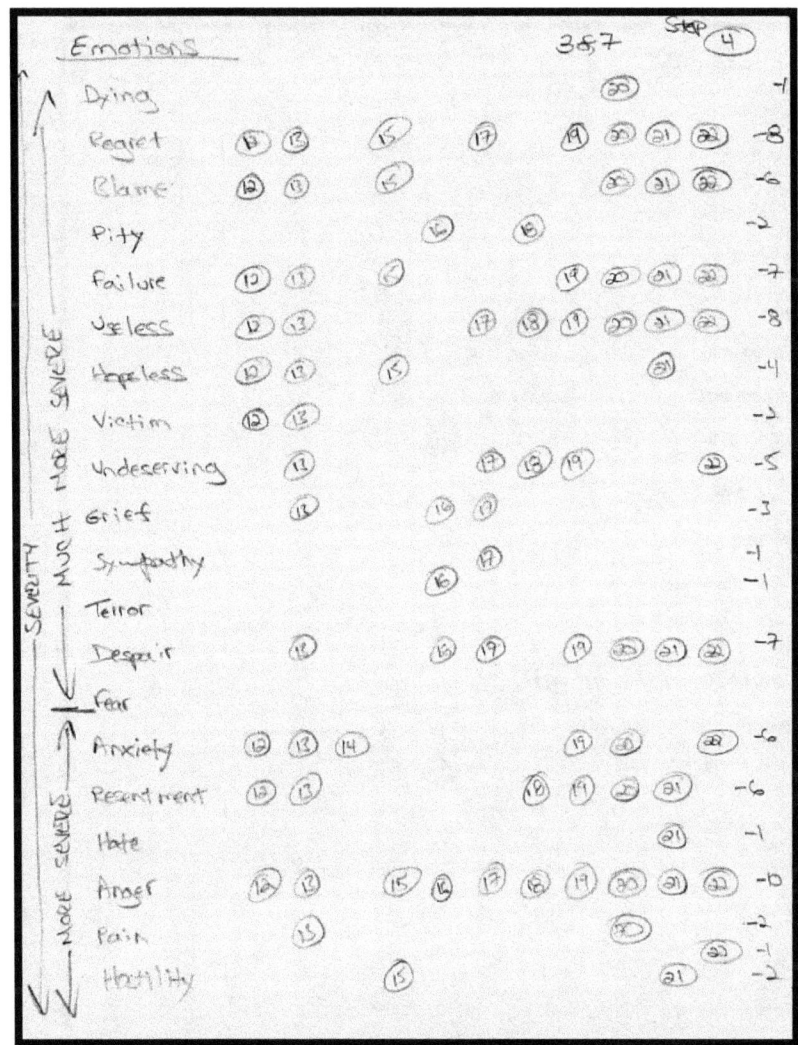

Figure 13c. My example influence matrix.

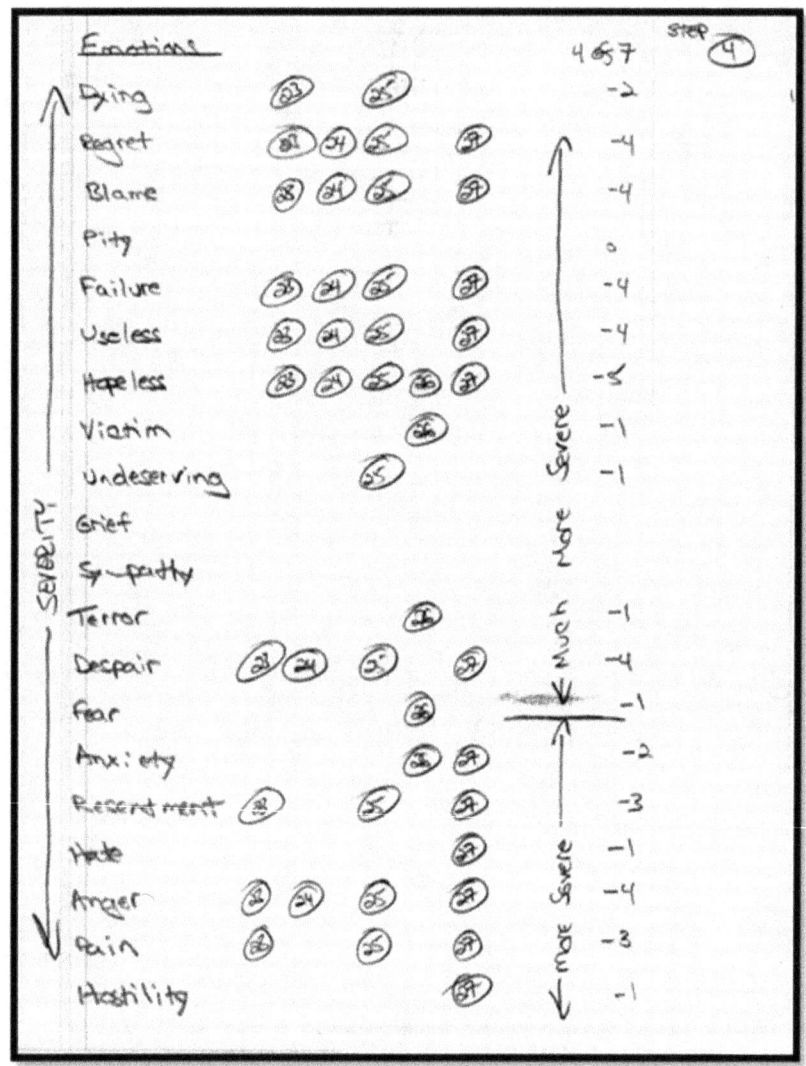

Figure 13d. My example influence matrix.

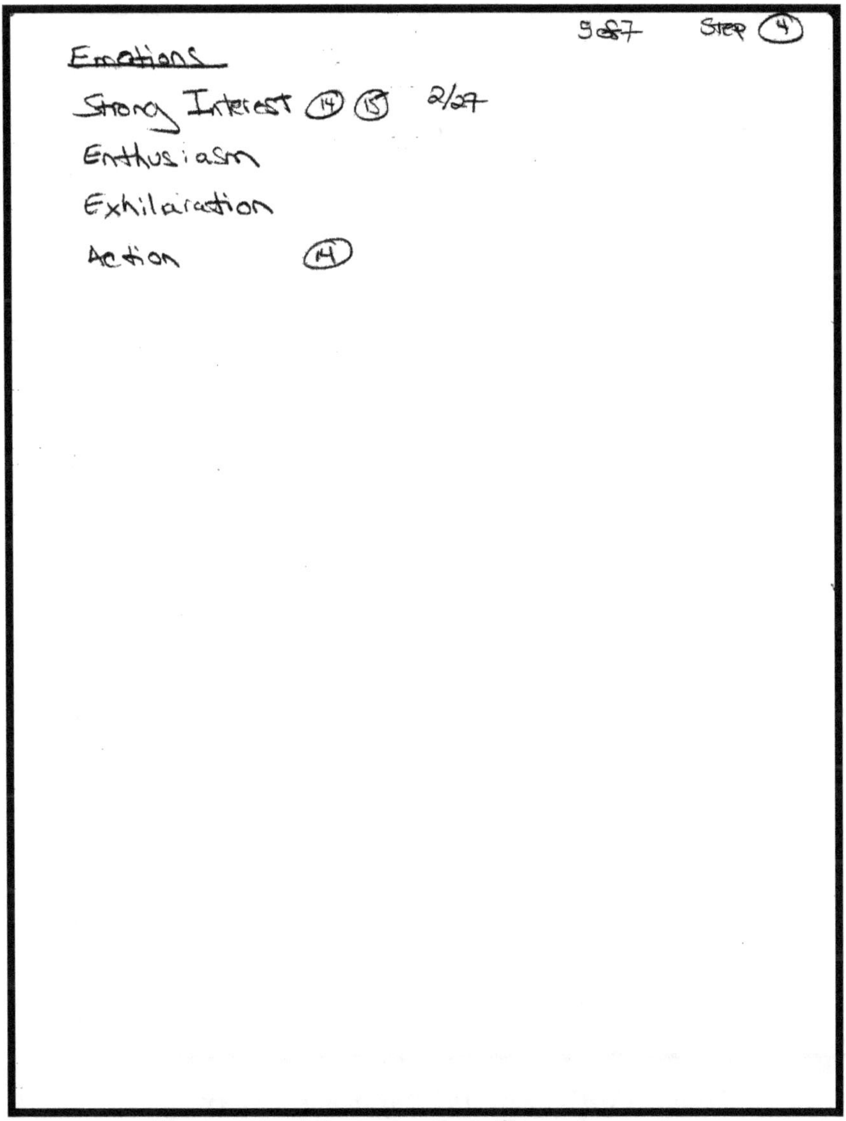

5 of 7
Step 4
Emotions
Strong Interest 14 15 2/27
Enthusiasm
Exhilaration
Action 14

Figure 13e. My example influence matrix.

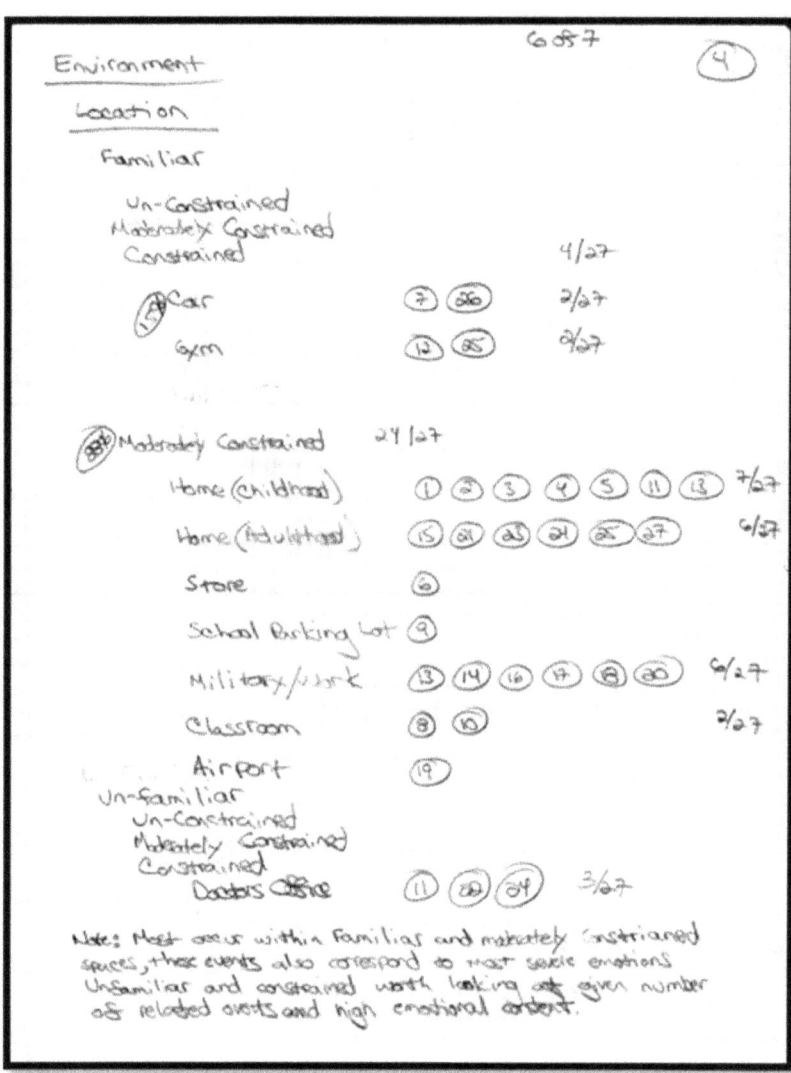

Figure 13f. My example influence matrix.

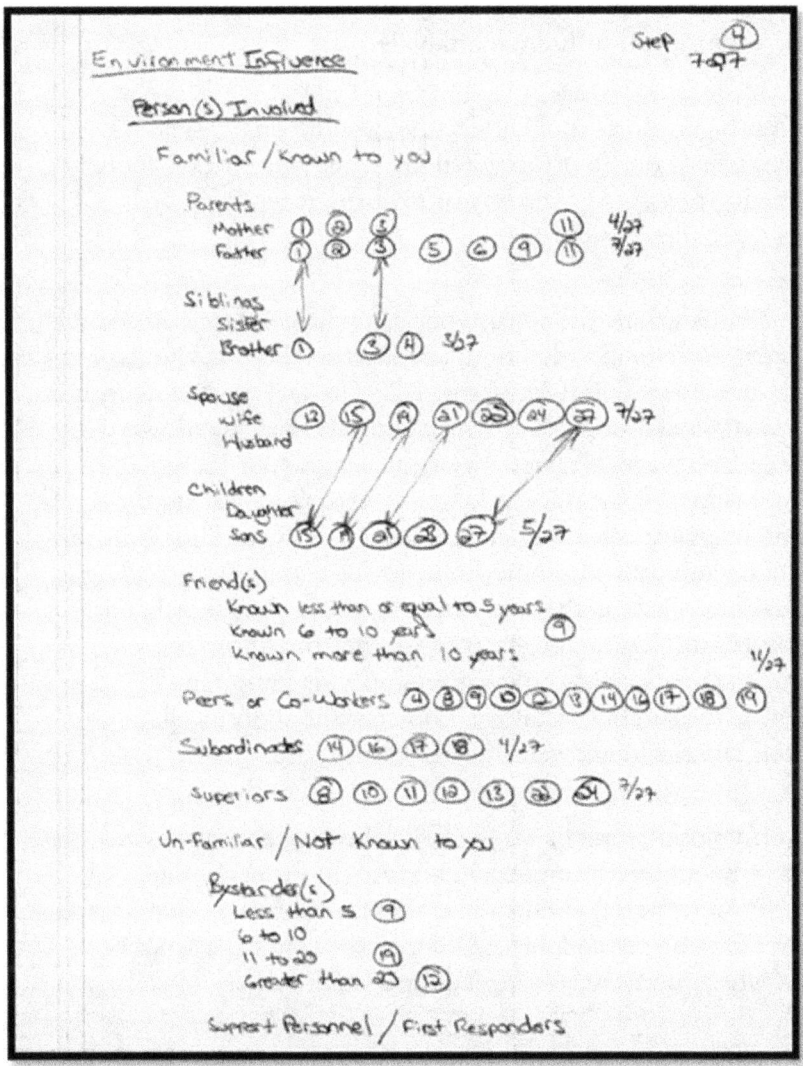

Figure 13g. My example influence matrix.

Step 4.A. Duration influence analysis.

Start with Figure 13a. You'll notice the heading on my sketch is duration, one of our four top tiered influence categories. I thought it interesting to assess how many of my experiences matched various categories of time.

This is where our consistency can pay off. Recall, I used the same terms to reference duration; less than an hour, 1-2 hours, 3-4 hours, 1 week, less than 12 months, 1-2 years, 3-4 years, and greater than 4 years in duration. Place your duration shorthand down the side of a blank piece of paper. Now go back to your Experience Decompositions. As you walk down the experience list start to populate that clean sheet of paper that contains your duration short hand. If all goes well you should start to see patterns or grouping begin to develop along the row extending form your shorthand. Congratulations! You've begun your journey out of the fog! Recognizing the fact that time has an impact is important. Remember the sun burn analogy. Look for the short dwell durations and the long dwell and reflect on those.

If you can, create a three rows below your durations analysis; Childhood, Young Adult, and Adult. From the data you collected resort the experiences into these three rows. What do you see now? Do you see a pattern? Did most of your experiences happen when you were a child? Young Adult? Adult?

I use the below ages for consistency purposes:

Childhood = 0 to 12
Young Adult = 13 to 19
Adulthood = 20 and older

With my own data I could see a pattern of experiences where they were either very short dwells or longer dwells. By placing a circle horizontally with the corresponding number from our chronological list we can also get a sense of when in time these experiences occurred relative to each other.

The fractions you see penciled in on the right are simple ratios. I wanted to understand out of all my experiences what the percentages would look like relative to the common durations. I penciled in some observations at the bottom of Figure 13a which gives you a sense on how I looked at this information as it was revealed to me at the time.

I have provided another way you may like to look at the influence of duration on your experiences. This figure is included in Appendix B-3 and is labeled, *Another way to look at duration and time.*

Step 4.B. Emotion analysis.

The remaining figures, Figures 13b through 13g, graphically depict my applicable influence factors paired against our experience. Think of the examples provided as a one to many relationship. A single influence factor is being evaluated with multiple experiences.

Just as demonstrated how we connected the influence factor of duration (or time) in the previous step, we will do the same here using the emotion factor. We'll look through our Experience Decompositions and identify those emotions so that we'll end up with a single sight picture of a specific emotion paired to a set of experiences.

First we'll want to identify the emotions that you identified in Step 3.B. Now go through your experiences, write down the emotions that you associated with your set of experiences. Order the emotions, without duplications, from most severe to least severe on a fresh piece of paper. Use Figure 9 to aid yourself in the ordering of the emotions. Remember, the emotions listed in Figure 9 are ordered from severe at the bottom to least severe at the top.

Once you have a list, on order, go back to your Decompositions. Place the experience in the same row that corresponds to the emotion. It's useful to go one experience at a time. It may take more paper but try to keep your experiences in a column running down the page. If it is done this way the effect is telling in two dimensions. I'll go into more detail in the following paragraphs.

Once you've completed this step you will have multiple emotion analysis pages. This is a good time to put the pencil down, clear off the writing area for a second, and place those emotion matrix pages down side by side. You should have the sheets so that each edge is butted up next to the other creating one long emotion matrix sketch. Lying the pages out in this manner provided me with a wealth of knowledge about myself. You'll notice on the left side of the page I made some annotations relative to the severity of the emotions listed. I also developed ratios so I could easily identify which specific emotional influence was most felt. By numbering the circles the way we did you can now use the matrix to identify (fairly easily) when in time the emotion(s) were experienced.

Now we can begin to draw connections between influences, events, and even time.

Step 4.C. Environment (Location and People) influence analysis.

We are now on our second to last influence category. When I developed this process, environment was not as mature of a factor as I have it listed now. I believe this to be an advantage of the process. The sketches included in this book reflect some of my earlier work, again, they do not represent the more mature model described earlier. The framework is extensible....So, extend it.

Our approach to environment will be similar to the previous categories. Figure 13f provides an example, again, this does not represent the more detailed outline we discussed earlier in Section 3, step 3.C.

Ask yourself, "Where did the majority of the experiences fall? Were they in familiar or unfamiliar surroundings? What were the weather conditions? Did a majority occur during a storm? Isolated conditions?

As you evaluate the "people" portion of the category ask some simple questions, "Was it crowded?" "Was it predominantly unfamiliar people involved? "Were they relatives?" "Friends?" Once again you are looking for groupings that possibly be a leading indicator, an indicator that just might trigger an ah ha moment.

Step 4.D. Personality influence analysis.

Hopefully this is becoming easier. I realized after creating my initial sketches and writing my waypoints in the first book, there was a personality contribution that I had missed. My very persona had played a role in my experiences. There's no doubt in my mind that what makes up "Me" influenced the experience outcome. It influenced the outcome as much as the duration, time, and environment had.

My sense is you will not have much to analyze here with regard to significant change. If you do, that may be worth reflecting on. Ask yourself, "Did my personality attribute change over time? If it did, "What experiences surround the change (look at experiences to the left and right within the time domain)?" It may also be worth looking at other hierarchy influences. "Was there a significant influence in those surrounding experiences?" "What were the surrounding experiences when it changed?"

The beauty is you have all the information at your fingertips. You can ask all the questions you want, you have the data about YOU right in front of YOU.

Section 4 Summary.

This section has further developed the rough sketches we developed in Section 3. Specifically, we have developed a process to analyze an experience relative to a host of contributing factors. By pivoting the data from Section 3 we found some unique perspectives. Perspectives that when looked at in total provide us a knowledge. Knowledge of our experiences, but even more importantly, knowledge of ourselves. In the Chapter that follows we will explore this data using a couple of unique concepts. Concepts with origins steaming as far back as the 2nd millennia and the 1800's.

Section 5: Generating a Seurat Experience Matrix.

You probably wondered how Seurat would finally fit in, and here he is. I began my first book considering my life experiences as waypoints. This made logical senses to me seeing as I was trained as a Navigator the Navy. It seemed to be a natural metaphorical fit. I can't imagine anything better resembling the loneliness and isolation one feels with severe depression than the imagery of a Tall Sailing ship of old, floating aimlessly in the fog, perilously close to a rocky shore line, as a single crew member contemplates his own fate. It just seemed to fit.

In my previous book I reflect on how Georges Seurat almost didn't make the cut, the only reason the section about Georges Seurat stayed in the book was due to my wife. She liked it. Having been married for 25 years I wasn't going to tell her no. I proceeded with using my waypoints and she got to see the section remain in the book, all of us were happy. When you read the *Journey* books, and I encourage you to do so, remember the waypoint is used interchangeably with a "Seurat dot".

Step 5.A. Generating a Seurat Experiences Matrix.

Use a blank piece of paper, a piece of graphing paper may be most helpful. Begin by numbering the page on the left side from top to bottom. I simply restated my earlier chronological list here. A simple circle with the number in the center will be fine. Refer to Figure 14, *My Seurat Experience Matrix* for some idea of what I mean as we go through these steps.

Step 5.B. Label the columns with our top tier influence categories.

Label the columns of the page as I did in Figure 14. I used shorthand notation on mine such as "D" for duration, "E" for emotion, "Ev" for environment, and "Me" for the personality trait.

Step 5.C. Identify lifetime phases (if applicable).

Now that we have our chronological listing and headings across our page lets go ahead and place a solid line across the page identifying the following: Childhood, Young Adult, and Adulthood. Once again, I used the following for my definition of these phases (refer to Figure 14 as an example):

Childhood   = 0 to 12
Young Adult   = 13 to 19
Adulthood   = 20 and older

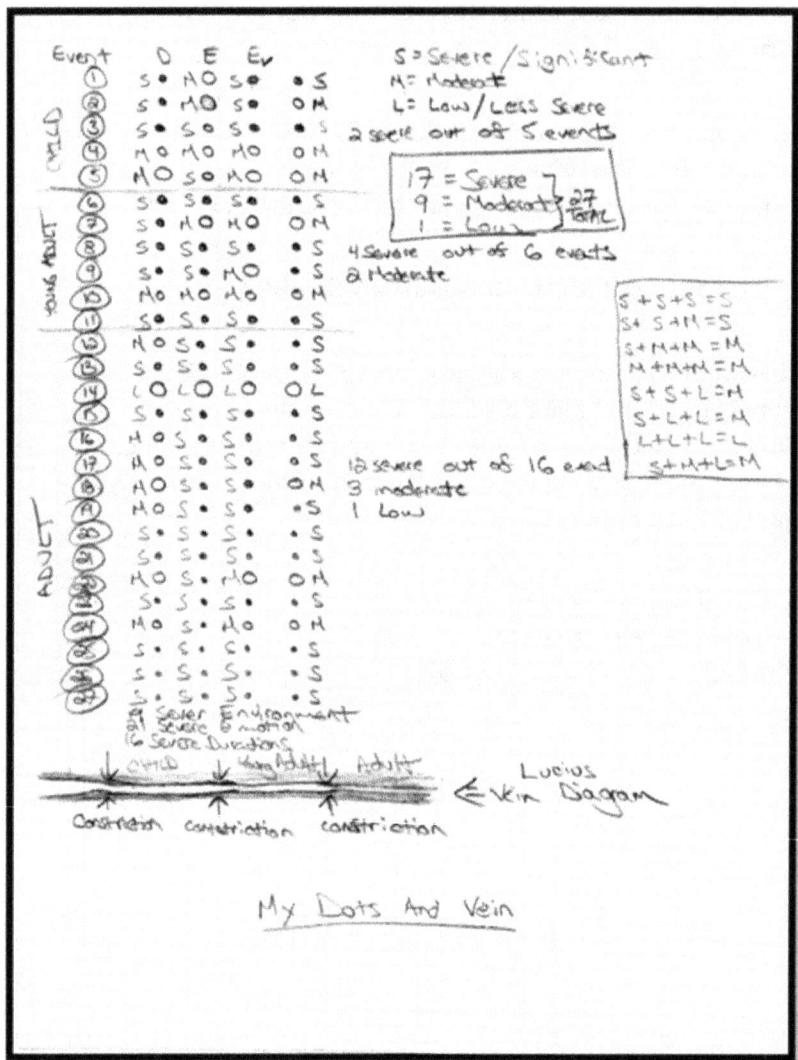

Figure 14. My Seurat Experience Matrix

Step 5.D. Identify contribution of influences.

Here's the really interesting portion of the process. Before we begin, we'll need to once again agree on some definition of terms.

I developed three categories which I felt met my needs to define the contribution a specific influence area had on my experience:

Severe / Significant, Moderate / Medium, and Low / Less.

This is where we have to agree. These are subjective terms, I get it. For the purposes of our process these three vague categories will suffice. Remember, I used the *KISS* principle throughout the process.

Now, with a clear mind (take some of those deep breaths) let's look at our first experience. It helped me to refer back to my experience decompositions, Figures 12a through 12d.

Before we get started. We'll need to agree on a standard annotation for the three influence contribution categories. This is important. The visual effect will be telling once you complete this matrix. Recall the analogy of the human vein and the relationship we derived to a *Lucius Emotional Vein*. We discussed how a human vein can become constricted. If the vein is fully constricted it could mean stroke or worse, death. We're now going to going to aggregate our influence areas into a diameter of a circle. For simplicity I used three sizes. I also used three sizes because I had spare change in my desk drawer. I had a quarter, a nickel, and a dime. I guess you say this writing cost me 40 cents and five years of living with severe depression, what a deal.

I used a small dot to represent a severe or significant contribution (think constricted vein = badness), a medium size circle or dot to represent a moderate contribution (think somewhat constricted = moderately constricted), and a large circle or dot to represent less or low contribution for a particular influence category (think near normal or slight constriction).

Now go back to our graph paper. Once you have a good idea again of the experience look at the column headings one by one. Ask yourself, "How significant was Duration to my experience relative to the other three influences?"

1. Was duration a significant contributing factor? If so make a small dot in the column along the same row as the experience.
2. Was duration a moderately contributing factor relative to the other three? If so make a medium size dot.
3. Was duration less of a factor of the four? If it was, place a larger dot or circle in the corresponding column and row.

Now move onto the next column still assessing the same first experience. Ask yourself the same questions as above except this time we will substitute the emotion(s) influence.

It is also just fine to use the same size dot as you had done for the previous influence. That would just signify to me you felt the two to be of the same significance.

You'll repeat this process using both environment and personality.

Once completed go on to the next experience. Ask yourself the same questions and continue to fill in your Seurat Experience Matrix.

Section 6. Analyzing the Seurat Experience Matrix.

As the teacher would say, "PENCILS DOWN!" We've done a lot of writing and sorting on various bits of information up to this point. A boss of mine once told me after sending him a lengthy and technically detailed email, "Freddie, all data no knowledge."

What he was telling me was, I provided a bunch of data but failed to reason on it and provide the so what. It's easy for us to regurgitate information; it's another thing to extract meaningful knowledge from the information.

We now have our matrix boxes completed with our Seurat Experience Dots and just like the painting, *Sunday Afternoon on the Island of La Grande Jatte,* we can take a step back, look at our dots, and begin to reason on what we see. What knowledge can we glean? We'll dive into a few approaches in the steps below.

Step 6. Seurat Experience Dots.

We have a consolidated picture of our dots. Take a look and see what conclusions or connections your Seurat Experience Matrix may be telling you. Do you have a lot of tight, small circles?

Remember; smaller = constrained = bad.

Do you have groupings of smaller circles relative to a period in your life, say childhood?

As you answer these questions look at the circle with the number in the center. That circle represents an influential point in time of your life.

In Figure 14, *My Seurat Experience Dot Matrix*, I placed a small key on the right hand side of my sketch. It shows a series like these: s - s - s = s or, s - s - m = s. I'm using a shorthand. I wanted to understand the overall severity of the experience so I developed the shorthand. It is simply a combination of influence factors all assumed to be equally weighted. This method allowed me to evaluate the number of severe, moderate or low experiences I may have had. Using the periods of my life as identified by the solid line, I can also determine in which period these significant events occurred (think of it as concentration point).

If you begin to discover themes or common connections it may be advisable to reflect back on the individual influence sketches we developed previously. These might yield some additional interesting results.

Remember the approach I am describing here is not scientific. This method is intended to simply provide an individual another method, another tool for self-reflection and evaluation.

My hope is simply that you find value in the process. I strongly urge you to take your findings and notes to your professional clinician.

I utilized my notes from the book as discussion topics during my time with the therapist. There was significant benefit having someone listen and aid in the interpretation of the information.

Bottom-line, the information you just collected on yourself is an excellent way to start the next talk therapy session.

Chapter 3. The Lucius Experience Vein.

I commented on *Lucius Annaeus Seneca the Younger*, the philosopher who lived in 4BC, was an advisor to Emperor Nero, and who was forced to commit suicide because he was considered involved in a possible assassination attempt.

He was also the one that I discovered the following quote by:

> *What is the highway to freedom? Any vein in your body*
> *Lucius Annaeus Seneca the Younger*

It has taken me nearly five years, and I believe I finally developed an interpretation of Lucius' writing.

Over the past many years I've taken the quote and turned it on its head. I thought to myself, "Hey, why can't an experience be captured and turned into something more tangible?" We live in a very "stuff" orientated society. We like our things. Why couldn't I take an experience and turn it into something.

We think of experiences and emotions as intangible items, unseen to the naked eye. You can't walk up to someone and ask, "Pardon me. Can I have a pound of fear please?" or "Pardon, can I have a half dozen of those experiences over there please?" This analogy is akin to the insurance commercial that displays insurance as boxes on a shelf. Just like insurance experiences are difficult to capture in box form.

I wanted to create something that could be viewed much like what we see on the following page in Figure 15, *Portion of the human vein structure.*

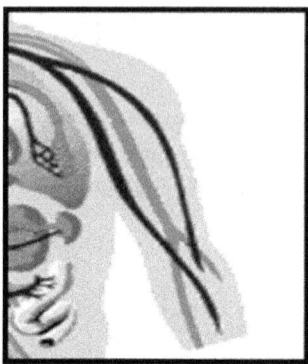

Figure 15. Portion of the human vein structure.

A look at the figure above reveals our "human-ness". Literally, showing us the pathways of our blood, that which makes us alive. That vein structure you see. That vein structure has been with you since birth. The structure of veins has grown with you, over time.

Look down at your forearm and make a fist several times. Watch as the veins begin to come to the surface. That is you. If you could travel through those arteries, what would you see? For some, they would be nice cylindrical tubes with blood flowing freely and uninterrupted. Unfortunately for some, you may have a different picture. One showing points of constriction or narrowing of the vein due to the build of plaque along the vein walls. What happens when that plaque builds and builds? If untreated, the vein becomes narrower, and narrower. The blood struggles to make its way through the body. If the blood is completely cut off, this could lead to stroke, and or death. Not a very nice outcome especially when there are ways to treat this sort of thing. There's medication, there's life style changes, etc. In some severe cases there's even a medical procedure called angioplasty that can widen those narrowed and constricted arteries. Please keep these thoughts in your mind as we proceed.

What if you could take an experience, turn it into something visible to the naked eye, just like that vein in your arm. What if we had a way to depict our experiences in three dimensions? Like that artery we just described.

Instead of an experience being some nebulous unseen thing; what if I say we can give an experience range, depth, and even color. In a very rudimentary way we can take an experience and visually look at it. If we have multiple experiences, we can knit them together. We can journey through and like the doctor conducting an angioplasty, we can see points of constriction. Points where the walls be begin to get tighter and smaller, cutting of the flow. What if we call this object our Emotional Vein? So maybe, just maybe, what Lucius was trying tell me was that freedom can be sought not by cutting through your biological vein, but by exploring the emotional veins that run through all of us.

This Chapter is devoted to discovering how we can create our own Lucius Emotional Vein.

Section 1. The highway to freedom.

I can't tell you how many times I simply wanted a cure for my depression. I wanted a magical pill that would make me better, make me normal again. I recall watching the television and seeing those commercials for testosterone deficiency. I even went as far as to Google the symptoms. I looked at the various medical websites and of course, go through the list of symptoms. I'd say to myself, "Yes. I have that one. Yes have that one. YES! I have that one as well. Awesome!" I remember feeling excited, "THIS IS IT! I have testosterone deficiency! YES! YES!" All I could imagine were those commercials. The cure for the disease was something I could just rub under my arm pits and I'd be cured. My wife would have her "old Todd back" once again. My life would be back to normal.

I went as far as to make an appointment with my Urologist. I needed a follow-up from a prostate thing I had a couple of years back so the timing worked out perfectly. I went to the appointment, got through the prostrate piece of the exam, pulled my pants back up and asked the doc, "So doc. I'm feeling kind of sluggish and tired all the time. Do you think I have a testosterone deficiency?" There should have been a drum roll in the background. I was anxious, very anxious. He looked at me, "Well, we can check. I'll put in a lab to have it checked." "YES, YES! I knew it. I knew I had it." The doc might as well put the scrip in for the medication now. It's as good as done. Just give me the stuff to put under my pits now and I'll be happily on my way.

The doctor left the office, moments later the nurse raps on the door. The nurse enters the small exam room carrying a small blue colored plastic bin. The bin was filled with all the tools she needed to take my blood; test tubes, rubber bands, and oh ya, even more test tubes.

The nurse sat the bin down on the desk and pulled out a wide blue rubber band and wrapped it tightly around my arm. It only took seconds before I could see the veins start to protrude from under my skin. I squeezed my hand into a fist several times just to speed up the process.

I thought for just a split second about Lucius. How did he do it? How did he kill himself? Did he slit both wrists? Did he have to press very hard? Were his arms submerged in water? I read somewhere that the stoics had bath tubs for just such a task. What did it feel like as his lifeblood left his body?

Several years ago, I had a procedure done that caused me to lose about half of my volume of blood. I recall nearly passing out one evening while my wife instinctively reached around my body to ease my collapsing body. I was light headed, woozy, and fatigued all at the same time. Did Lucius feel the same way? Is that he felt as he bleed out? A slow and forever slumber.

With a couple of fingers the nurse taps on my arm, right below where the tightened band. Her tapping on my arm causes my attention to refocus on what she was about to do. I looked down at my arm as the nurse holds the need perpendicular to the floor. The needle slips effortlessly through the tissue of my skin. She moves the needle under my skin. First a slight bit to the right, then a bit to the left. She applies a bit more pressure. My vein tries not to cooperate. The vein rolls away from the needle's sharpened tip. The vein knows it's being intruded upon. The nurse continues to work the needle back and forth under the skin of my arm. A sharp pain builds, but for some odd reason, I like it. I don't want the pain to stop.

The nurse finally captures what she has been looking for, my blood. She reaches into the blue plastic bin and pulls out a vial and pushes it onto the back side of the needle, now inserted into my arms vein. The pressure of her hand pushing down on the back side of the needle felt good, in an odd sort of way.

Like a rush of water out of a tap faucet, a thick red liquid fills the tube. My blood rushes out of its home into a new resting place. The blood fills the tube, she reaches around my arm, and releases the band that had been constricting my arm. She places her other hand just above the needle and slowly pulls the needle from the inside of my arm. At the same time, she presses a piece of gauze down where the blood was once freely flowing. Oh Lucius, if y I could have found my highway to freedom this day.

Two weeks go by, I have yet to hear back from the nurse or doctor about the results from the lab. It felt like I was waiting on the delivery of my first born. I just couldn't wait any longer. I picked up the phone in my office and dialed the doctor's office. "Hello, doctor XX's office. How can I help you?" Anxious to get the words out, "Hmm, this is Mr. Kruder. I was in a couple of weeks back and the doctor ordered some blood work. I'd just like to know if the results arrived yet." Drum roll please. The voice on the other end says, "Mr. Kruder.....Ah yes. Just a second while I find your chart. .... Here it is…... This was for a low testosterone, correct?" I'm sitting on the edge of my seat and just wanted to shout back, "YES!   YES! While thinking to myself, "Please just give me the results."

There was a pause on the other end of the phone, "It was negative. The levels were fine. Is that all you needed today?" You could have heard the proverbial pin drop in my office. I felt like I wanted to throw the phone across the office. I couldn't believe it. "How could it be negative? I had all the god damn symptoms. I need my cure!"

I hung up the phone. I starred at it for a long time, it took me a while to absorb the news. "I didn't have my cure. Until I do, my journey will continue in the fog."

Section 2. Constructing a Lucius Emotional Vein.

Why did I bore you with such a story in the previous section? Well, there are a couple of reasons. First, the story describes to you how profoundly my thoughts were impacted by Lucius. The second reason, the vein Lucius referred to in his quote allowed me consider the concept of an *emotional vein.*

When I watched my blood pour into the vial, I pondered the quote one more time, "If Lucius was referring to an emotional vein the quote may look much differently:"

What is the highway to freedom? Any emotional vein in your body.

"What components might make-up this vein? What could I use to give the vein the range and depth I desired?" I know it's difficult to imagine and it's difficult to take the time and create these sketches, but it is possible. Figure 16 on the following page labeled, *My Lucius Vein Structure,* is a simple representation of my chronological experiences within a *Lucius Emotional Vein* construct.

This is not a scientific approach, I get it. What this construct does do, is provide a means to view my experiences as a whole. It is the acknowledgment that my experiences were real, they had an effect, and they contributed to defining who I am today.

My experiences, my memories, they run through me like the very blood that runs through my veins today. Collectively they form *My Lucius Vein Structure.* In the upcoming pages we will step through this process together.

Section 3. Creating the vein structure.

We'll run through a demonstration of how you can sketch your own Lucius emotional vein. This is a good time to grab those coins I mentioned earlier. Staying with the *KISS* philosophy, I simply used a dime, a nickel, and a quarter. You certainly can use a stencil or some other device that gives you the desired outcome.

It's a good idea to start fresh with a new sheet of paper. At this point I definitely prefer to use the graphing paper. I'm not so good with drawing straight lines.

Set the Lucius Experience Matrix we created next to you for easy reference (Ref Figure 14). With the graph paper in the landscape position, sketch a quarter size circle on one end and parallel to the first circle make another on the far right hand side, this is where the graph paper helps ensure you are parallel with the first circle.

Now with a straight edge (a ruler is good to use here) connect the two circles with two straight lines running tangent to the tops and bottoms of the circumferences. As an example I provided my structure as a reference as Figure 16, *My Lucius Vein Structure* . How straight were your lines? It's ok, remember, we have erasers for just that purpose. The large circumference represents a normal sized vein, unconstructed. Think childhood before you started pounding back the fried fast foods out there.

Once you created the normalized vein lets place some timeline labels on it for reference points. The length of the vein will represent the minimum and maximum duration of your experiences (Ref Figure 12a). The left hand side will be the start of your first event while the right side will represent the completion of the last event on our chronological experience list in figure 7a and 7b. If you have a good feel for time go ahead and place a year marker at the left for the first and a year marker on the far right. Find the center and annotate it with the middle of the time period.

Now we have our basic vein structure drawn with a relative duration based on our experiences.

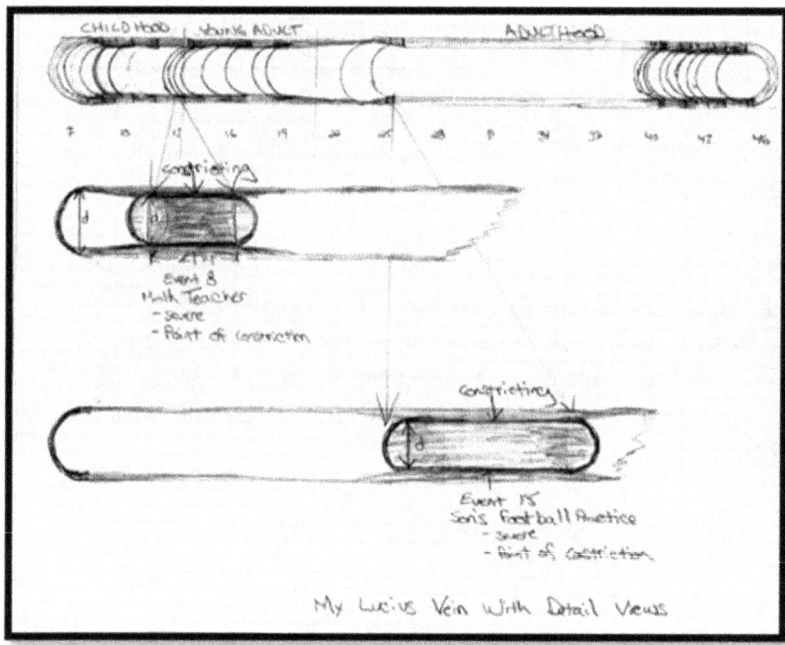

Figure 16. My Lucius Vein Structure.

Section 4. Filling in the Lucius Experience Vein.

Remember, the purpose behind this is to show how our emotional vein structure looks once we add those experiences we listed in previous steps.

Look at the Seurat experience matrix we developed. Look at the first event on the list. What was the overall severity we gave the experience? Was it an "S", "M", or an "L"? Depending on what it was use a corresponding circle. Remember the smaller circle represents a more severe experience = "S" in this case.

This is where it gets a bit tricky. This is far from scientific so bear with me. If, for example, your first event was severe. I would be using the dime sized circle representing the smallest of the three diameters. I'd place it at the beginning of my vein and trace it. Here's the really tough part. The length of the vein segment will be a ratio of the experience duration or time and the entire emotional vein length (think fractions of time). As long as you're consistent with your eyeballing it should be fine (Ref Figure 16).

You'll repeat the above steps for each event / experience on your experience matrix

Section 5. Analyzing the Lucius Experience Vein.

Congratulations, you now created your Lucius Experience Vein. Depending on the number of experiences and overall duration you should be able to discern varying diameters and lengths (Time Duration).

With the edge of your pencil go ahead now and fill in between the vein segments. Doing this allows you to get a better picture of your point of constriction. You should be able to see those segments along your experience vein that close in on itself. Much like a doctor performing angioplasty you can now look at your emotional vein and see where your life may have been constricted, pinched, or closed off. I would argue, those are significant points deserving of further reflection and discussion with your professional clinician. The therapist can assist you in some virtual angioplasty.

This result was in fact our overall purpose. Develop a step-by-step process of self-reflection that results in an enhanced understanding of your life experiences so that we can enhance traditional therapeutic plans available, strengthening the S.E.A.M.! Strengthening the S.E.A.M. so you do not end up like me, tearing yourself away from help prematurely, destroying yourself and your relationships in the process.

Remember, this is just a process. The results are highly dependent on the honest thought you put into it. If you feel you may have held back some influence or even an experience, I highly recommend simply adding those elements to your vein.

Remember

The quickest way to freedom and happiness is through your EMOTIONAL VEIN.

Chapter 4. Applications of the method.

I realize I have what they call, skin in the game and you expect nothing less from me if I didn't say, **"This is a game changer."** A game changer in the support to existing therapies of depression.

I postulate an individual considering suicide has only a small window of influence between the times the individual decides to commit the act to the actual time the act is carried out.

How many of us have heard the comment after discovering that someone has committed suicide, "How could he/she do that? What were they thinking?" The key word in this phrase is thinking. Why wouldn't that person pick up the phone and call a neighbor? Call a 1-800 suicide hotline number? Go to one of the many web sites that exist on the great World Wide Web? You're probably thinking, "Well, I would if that were me." And you likely would be right at this very moment. What if your state of mind was so chaotic with emotions? What if your head was in a deep, dark fog? What if you were in this fog and you were alone? Nowhere to go? What would you be thinking? Or should I say "What was he/she thinking?" My point is those persons considering suicide are likely not thinking logically as you are at this moment. Their logic is skewed by the depressive emotions or thoughts over a period of time. I can tell you help was the furthest thing from my mind. In fact, I specifically didn't want people to know I was hurting. I didn't want people to see my weakness. With the use of this method we can string a series of past experiences together, look through the emotional vein structure, and see where those constriction points exist.

A potential DoD application of this method could be used as a post mission assessment capability. Imagine soldiers first entering the service generate their emotional vein baseline. From the baseline, leadership may determine a particular individual's previous experience or exposure to dramatic events warrants assignment to job specialties not related directly to combat operations.

Imagine a convoy returning from an operation within a hostile environment. After the mission, those very same soldiers come back to the battalion HQ, sit down in front of a computer, and call up a S.E.A.M tool. The very same tool used when they entered the service. Each soldier enters a unique identification number and answers a series of questions. This software version of the tool could be capable of accepting multiple input sessions and possibly make assessments across input sessions and adding to the original experience vein construct.

The data could be archived until the soldier inputs another mission. During or after the deployment a brigade Surgeon can review a specific soldier's S.E.A.M. analysis. By review of the model results the doctor can determine if a particular individual is showing a statistical propensity toward depression and provide a recommended course of intervening behavioral health treatment.

The above could be just the beginning. With a large enough data set and tailoring of the variables this tool could be easily extended to the civil sector. The tool could be used in cases of child abuse, those who work in trauma centers, police, fire, and EMS personnel could all benefit.

Epilogue

I will end this book on a quote located at the bottom of this page. There is additional meaning behind this quote for me. Not long ago I found myself wallowing in self-pity. A shipmate of mine and friend sent me an email. I was struggling to find purpose. I wanted to help others who suffered from the same illness as I. I looked at various organizations and became despondent. None of them fit for me. They were all like putting pants on that were three or four sizes too big.

My wife and I looked to establish our own Non-Profit. I guess you can say we figured we'd make our own pair of pants. Well, as we did, we realized we needed a mission and goals. I instantly looked to my wife and said, "That's easy. We'll do peer-peer counseling." She looked at me for a bit and said, "I guess so. Don't you need training to do that sort of thing?" "I don't know. If we do, we'll get the training." So, we moved on with the Non-Profit. We matured the goals a bit and educated ourselves along the way. As we educated ourselves we discovered a plethora of Non-Profits all focused on provided counseling to Military and Veteran communities. We sat through a Transition program (cool word for those of us going to pasture, leaving the military). A fine young man stood up at the front of the classroom and said, "Hello Everyone. I'm from the Department of Veterans Affairs. Please take one of these handouts." He passed out a small trifold brochure. "If you open it you'll find the contact numbers for your Vet Centers." He immediately stated, "Add I don't mean veterinarian centers. The name is a bit off, I know. These are faculties run by the Department of Veterans Affairs and manned by volunteers. We provided counseling services…..We are located mostly nearby major military installations…." After he was done you could have heard all the air in my body escape like putting a needle in a balloon. He basically described everything we were going to try and do through the Non-Profit. Later that same month, my wife surfed the web and discovered a host of Non-Profits, again, doing the exact same thing. I looked at my wife of 25 plus years and said, "Honey, we're not going to do counseling." "Why's that Todd?" "Because it's easy." "What? I don't understand." "Listen. With so many Non-Profits all doing counseling it can only mean one thing. It's easy. We will do what is hard." "And that would be?" "We will attack the left side of the problem." "Ok, I give up. What do you mean?" "I mean. We will attempt to develop tools that focus on interceding. Focus on predicting the illness, catching it before it leads to suicide." "Ok genius. How do we go about that?" "Well, I don't know. Like I said, it's a tough problem. That's why we need to make it our focus, our goal."

Since that conversation occurred we established two companies. A Non-Profit, Lucius Seneca Wellness Group and a Companion For-Profit, Seurat Innovations, LLC. We developed a hybrid business model that leverages the strengths of each while maintaining a synergistic Social Enterprise look at the problem of depression. The two companies will attempt at doing that which is hard.

Our ultimate goal is the establishment of a Behavioral Health Retreat for Active Duty, Veterans, and their families who have been either diagnosed with or have been identified as at risk for depression. Imagine a multi acre retreat away from the hustle and bustle of everyday life. Surrounded by nature, surrounded by the devine. A chance to reconnect with one's self and their families. Imagine these vary same active duty members receiving permissive TDY with their plane tickets paid for through the Non-Profit. That is our ultimate focus.

When I realized just how hard this would be that shipmate I mentioned earlier sent me an uplifting email. The email contained a number of salient points. He closed the email with the below quote. A quote so fitting that I adopted it to our For-Profit company's mantra.

Some of the world's greatest feats were accomplished by people not smart enough to know they were impossible. -- Doug Larson

About the Author

Captain Kruder accumulated over 25 years of faithful and dedicated service to our Nation.

He graduated from Lewis University and commissioned in 1988. He was designated a Naval Flight Officer in 1989. He completed two tours of duty within the Fleet Air Reconnaissance community accumulating over 2000 hours flying numerous sorties in support of Fleet and National Reconnaissance Operations. In 1993, he attended the Naval Post Graduate School where he earned his Master of Science. In 1999, he transitioned to the Aerospace Engineering Duty Officer community where served over 15 years conducting engineering, acquisition, and test.

His personal decorations include the Legion of Merit, Bronze Star, Meritorious Service Medal (three awards), Navy Commendation Medal (three awards), Joint Achievement Medal and the Navy Achievement Medal (three awards).

In the fall of 2009, diagnosed with severe depression, he found himself in and out of various behavioral health therapeutic treatments during a five-year period. Each time he removed himself from therapy, the event was proceeded by a more devastating impact on his life.

My List   Step ①
                                                1 & 2

Math Teacher

My Father and the grocery Store

The VQ flight

The Brigade Surgeon

The Brigade remembrance ceremony

My parents argument about Divorce

The "run-in" on the school parking lot

The football practice and my father

The football practice and my son

over looking the CBQ balcony in Norfolk

Standing in my kitchen with a hand full of meds

My Welcome home

The night in my Jeep

The Marine Recruiter and MEPS

The achilles tendon and OCS

The drill team competition

The English class in High School

Stormy Nights as a child

The sergeants thank you

The wedding ring incident

Step 1, 1of 2

Appendix-A 1

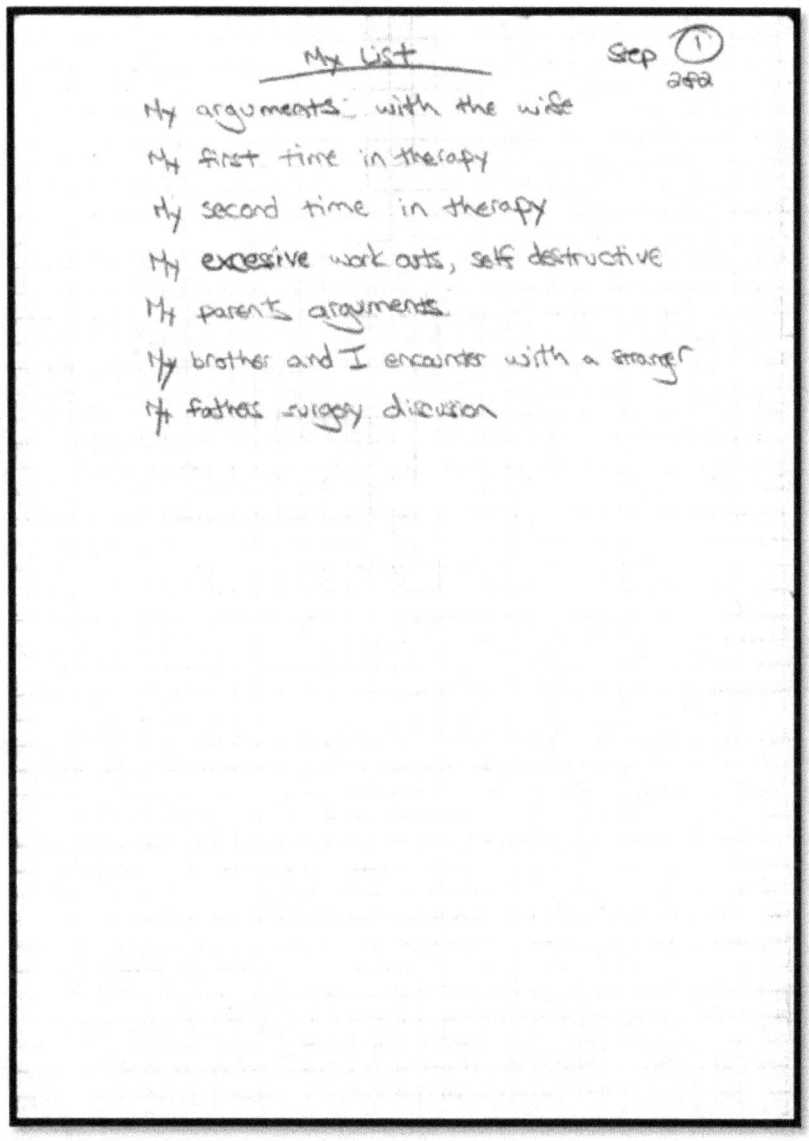

My List   Step ①
                                                2 of 2

My arguments with the wife
My first time in therapy
My second time in therapy
My excessive work outs, self destructive
My parents arguments
My brother and I encounter with a stranger
My fathers surgery discussion

Step 1, 2 of 2

Appendix-A   2

My Chronological List   Step ②
                                    1 &2

1. My parents arguments
2. Storming nights as a child
3. My parents argument about Divorce
4. My brother and I encounter with a Stranger
5. My fathers discussion of his surgery
6. My fathers incident in the grocery store
7. The grammar school football team practice
8. The grammer school Math teacher incident
9. The grammar school parking lot fight
10. The High school English room and teacher
11. The Marine Recruiter and NAS
12. The Drill Team incident
13. The achilles tendon injury and OCS
14. The VQ mission
15. My sons football practice incident
16. The brigade doctor suicide
17. The brigade memorials
18. The Sergeants thank you on the FOB
19. The welcome home

Step 2, 1 of 2

Appendix-A   3

My Chronological List   Step ②

2 of 2

20) The night at the CBQ in Norfolk

21) The arguments with my wife

22) The first time in therapy

23) The night in the kitchen with the meds

24) The second time in therapy

25) The excessive workouts and weight loss

26) The night in my Jeep on route 24

27) The wedding ring incident

Step 2, 2 of 2

Appendix-A   4

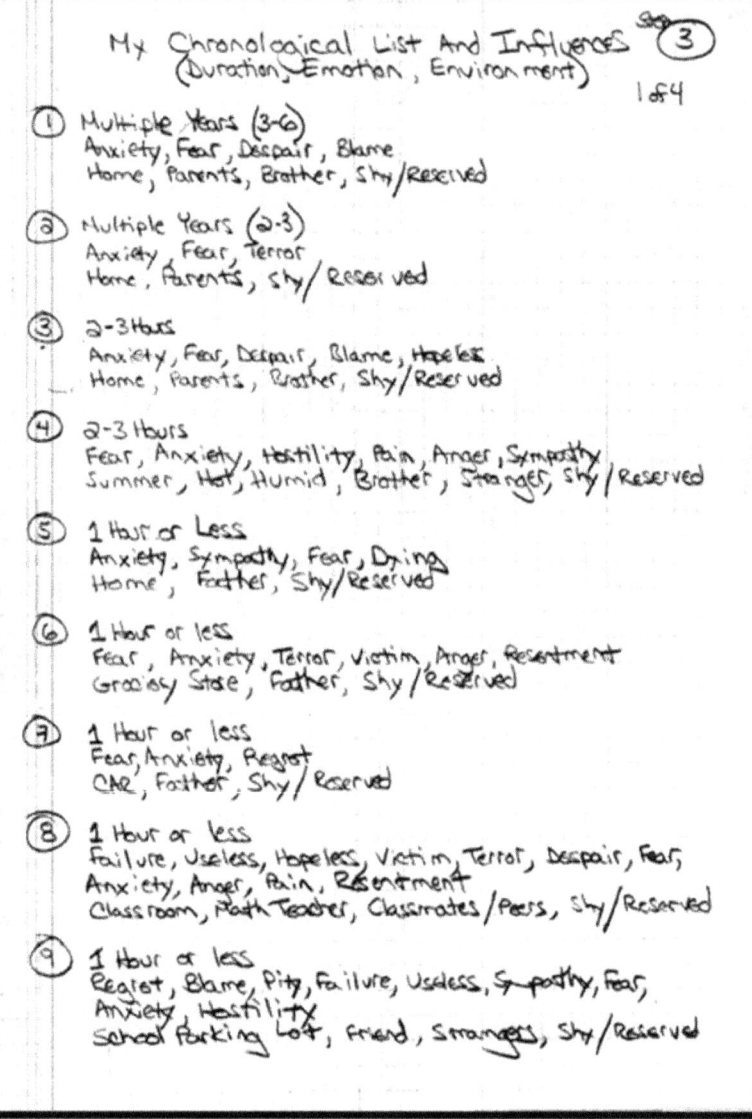

My Chronological List And Influences (Step 3)
(Duration, Emotion, Environment)
1 of 4

① Multiple Years (3-6)
Anxiety, Fear, Despair, Blame
Home, Parents, Brother, Shy/Reserved

② Multiple Years (2-3)
Anxiety, Fear, Terror
Home, Parents, Shy/Reserved

③ 2-3 Hours
Anxiety, Fear, Despair, Blame, Hopeless
Home, Parents, Brother, Shy/Reserved

④ 2-3 Hours
Fear, Anxiety, Hostility, Pain, Anger, Sympathy
Summer, Hot, Humid, Brother, Stranger, Shy/Reserved

⑤ 1 Hour or Less
Anxiety, Sympathy, Fear, Dying
Home, Father, Shy/Reserved

⑥ 1 Hour or less
Fear, Anxiety, Terror, Victim, Anger, Resentment
Grocery Store, Father, Shy/Reserved

⑦ 1 Hour or less
Fear, Anxiety, Regret
Car, Father, Shy/Reserved

⑧ 1 Hour or less
Failure, Useless, Hopeless, Victim, Terror, Despair, Fear,
Anxiety, Anger, Pain, Resentment
Classroom, Math Teacher, Classmates/Peers, Shy/Reserved

⑨ 1 Hour or less
Regret, Blame, Pity, Failure, Useless, Sympathy, Fear,
Anxiety, Hostility
School Parking Lot, Friend, Strangers, Shy/Reserved

Step 3, 1 of 4

Appendix-A   5

My Chronological List And Influences Step ③
(Duration, Emotion, Environment) 2 of 4

⑩ 1 Hour or less
Fear, Anxiety, Failure, Regret
High School Classroom, English Teacher, Classmates, Shy

⑪ 2-8 Months
Regret, Blame, Failure, Useless, Despair, Anxiety, Anger
Hostility
Home, MEPS, Parents, Doctors, Recruiter, Shy / Reserved

⑫ 2-4 Hours
Regret, Blame, Failure, Useless, Hopeless, Victim, Anxiety,
Anger, Resentment
College Gym, Drill Instructors, Team Members, Bystanders,
Shy/Reserved

⑬ 12-14 Months
Regret, Blame, Failure, Useless, Hopeless, Victim,
Undeserving, Grief, Despair, Anxiety, Resentment,
Pain, Anger
Home, College, ODS, Spouse/girlfriend, Peers, Drill
Instructors, Doctors

⑭ 3-4 Hours
Anxiety, Exhilaration, Action, Strong Interest
Aircraft, Cold, Peers and Subordinates, Reserved

⑮ 1-2 Hours
Anger, Hostility, Strong Interest, Hopeless, Failure,
Blame, Regret
Home, Spouse (wife), Son, Reserved, Summer, Hot, on Duty

⑯ ~1 Week
Pity, Grief, Sympathy, Despair, Anger
FOB, On Active Duty, Brigade, Peers Subordinates, Reserved

Step 3, 2 of 4

Appendix-A 6

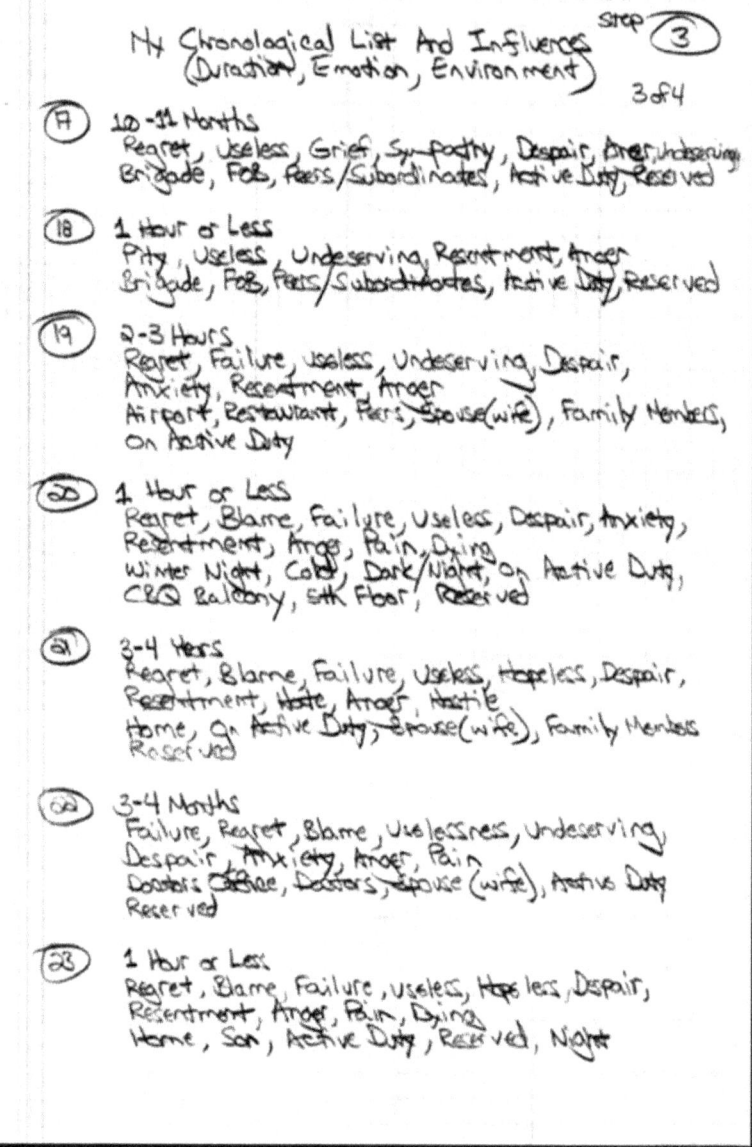

My Chronological List And Influences Step ③
(Duration, Emotion, Environment)
3 of 4

Ⓐ 10 - 11 Months
Regret, Useless, Grief, Sympathy, Despair, Anger, Undeserving
Brigade, FoB, Peers/Subordinates, Active Duty, Reserved

⑱ 1 Hour or Less
Pity, Useless, Undeserving, Resentment, Anger
Brigade, FoB, Peers/Subordinates, Active Duty, Reserved

⑲ 2-3 Hours
Regret, Failure, Useless, Undeserving, Despair,
Anxiety, Resentment, Anger
Airport, Restaurant, Peers, Spouse(wife), Family Members,
On Active Duty

⑳ 1 Hour or Less
Regret, Blame, Failure, Useless, Despair, Anxiety,
Resentment, Anger, Pain, Dying
Winter Night, Cold, Dark/Night, On Active Duty,
CBQ Balcony, 5th Floor, Reserved

㉑ 3-4 Hrs
Regret, Blame, Failure, Useless, Hopeless, Despair,
Resentment, Hate, Anger, Hostile
Home, On Active Duty, Spouse(wife), Family Members
Reserved

㉒ 3-4 Months
Failure, Regret, Blame, Uselessness, Undeserving
Despair, Anxiety, Anger, Pain
Doctors Office, Doctors, Spouse (wife), Active Duty
Reserved

㉓ 1 Hour or Less
Regret, Blame, Failure, Useless, Hopeless, Despair,
Resentment, Anger, Pain, Dying
Home, Son, Active Duty, Reserved, Night

Step 3, 3 of 4

Appendix-A 7

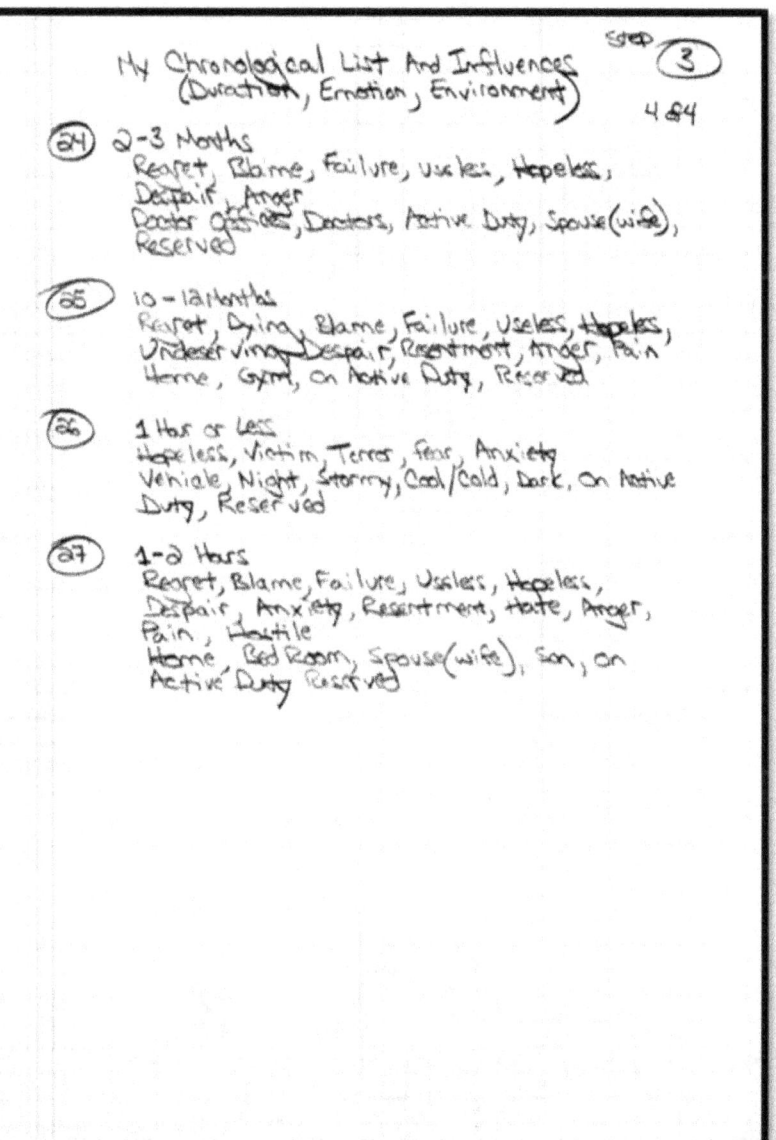

My Chronological List And Influences   step ③
(Duration, Emotion, Environment)   4 &4

24) 2-3 Months
Regret, Blame, Failure, Useless, Hopeless,
Despair, Anger
Doctor offices, Doctors, Active Duty, Spouse(wife),
Reserved

25) 10 - 12 Months
Regret, Dying, Blame, Failure, Useless, Hopeless,
Undeserving, Despair, Resentment, Anger, Pain
Home, Gym, On Active Duty, Reserved

26) 1 Hour or Less
Hopeless, Victim, Terror, Fear, Anxiety
Vehicle, Night, Stormy, Cool/Cold, Dark, On Active
Duty, Reserved

27) 1-2 Hours
Regret, Blame, Failure, Useless, Hopeless,
Despair, Anxiety, Resentment, Hate, Anger,
Pain, Hostile
Home, Bed Room, Spouse(wife), Son, on
Active Duty, Reserved

Step 3, 4 of 4

Appendix-A   8

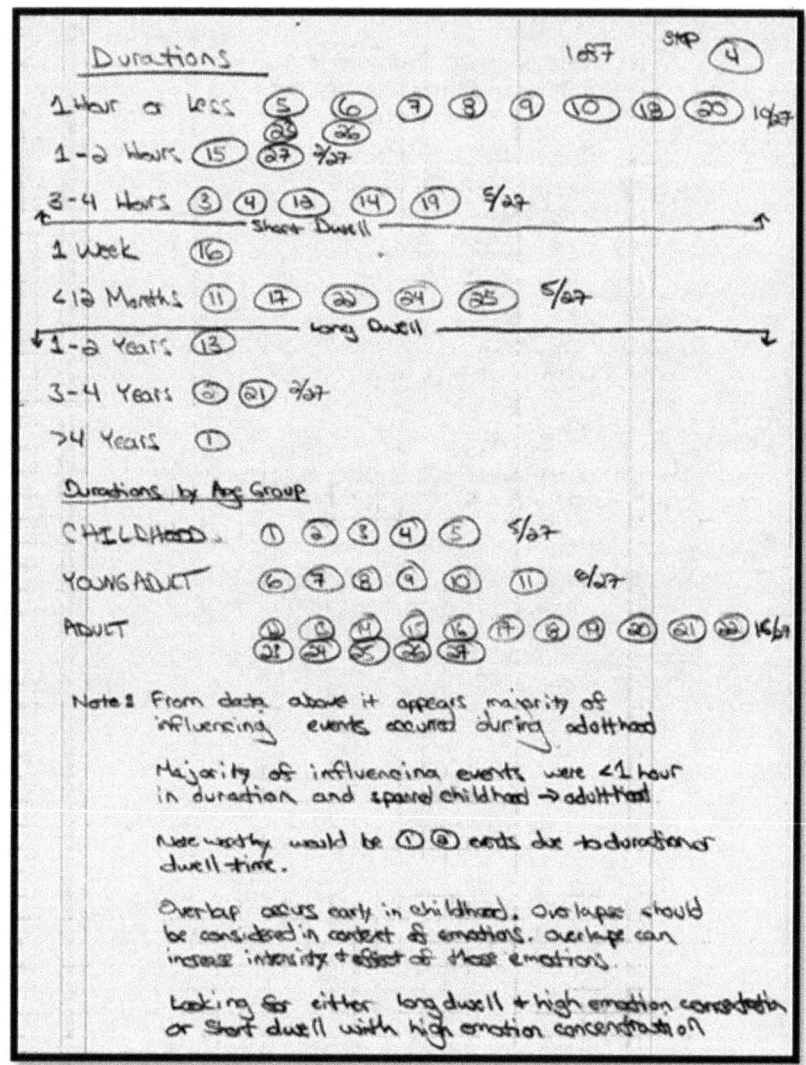

Step 4, 1 of 7

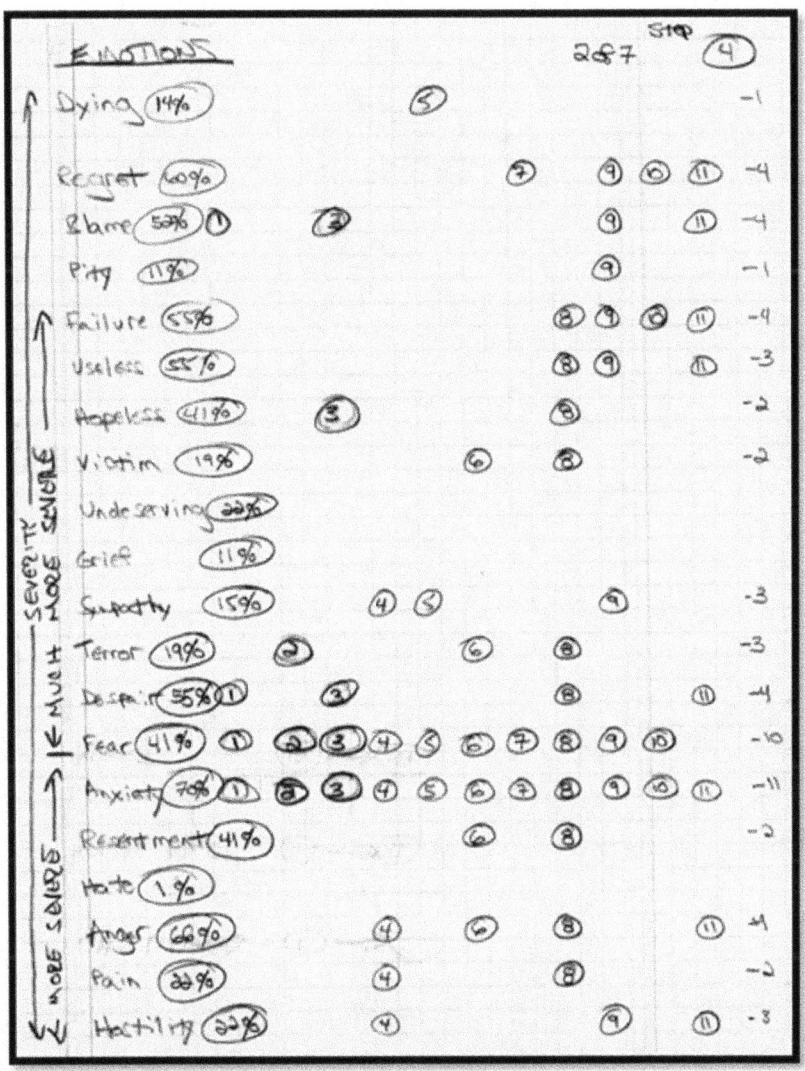

Step 4, 2 of 7

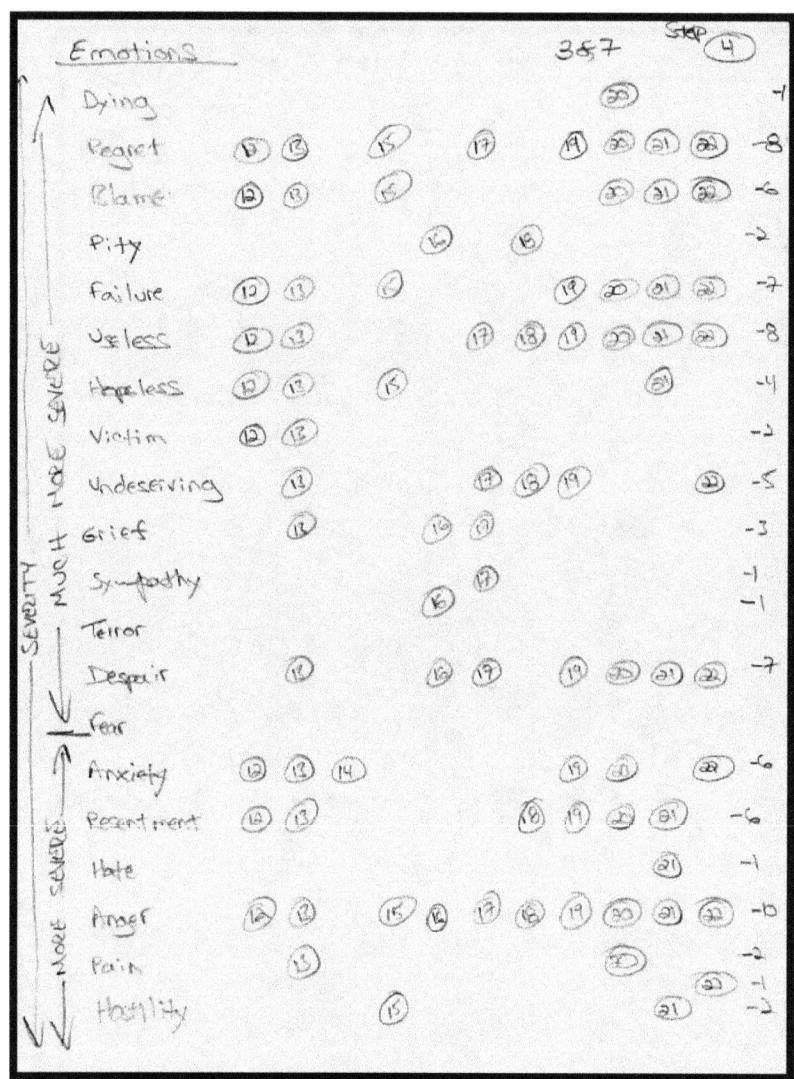

Step 4, 3 of 7

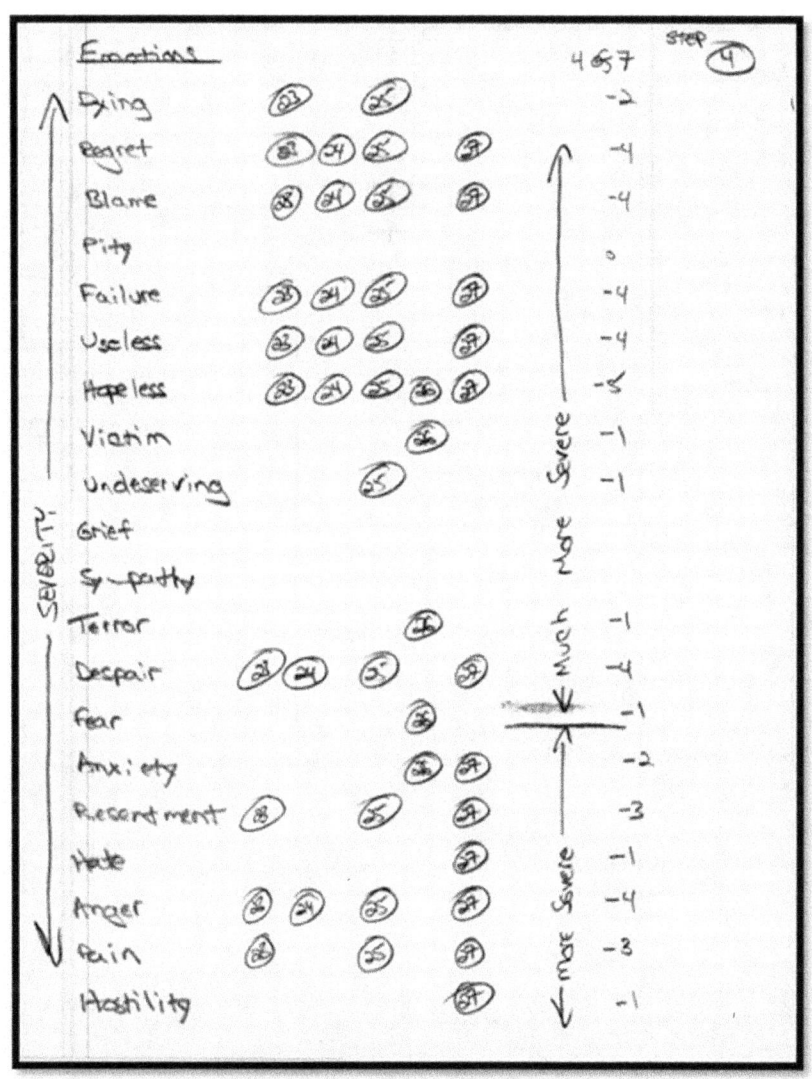

Step 4, 4 of 7

Appendix-A   12

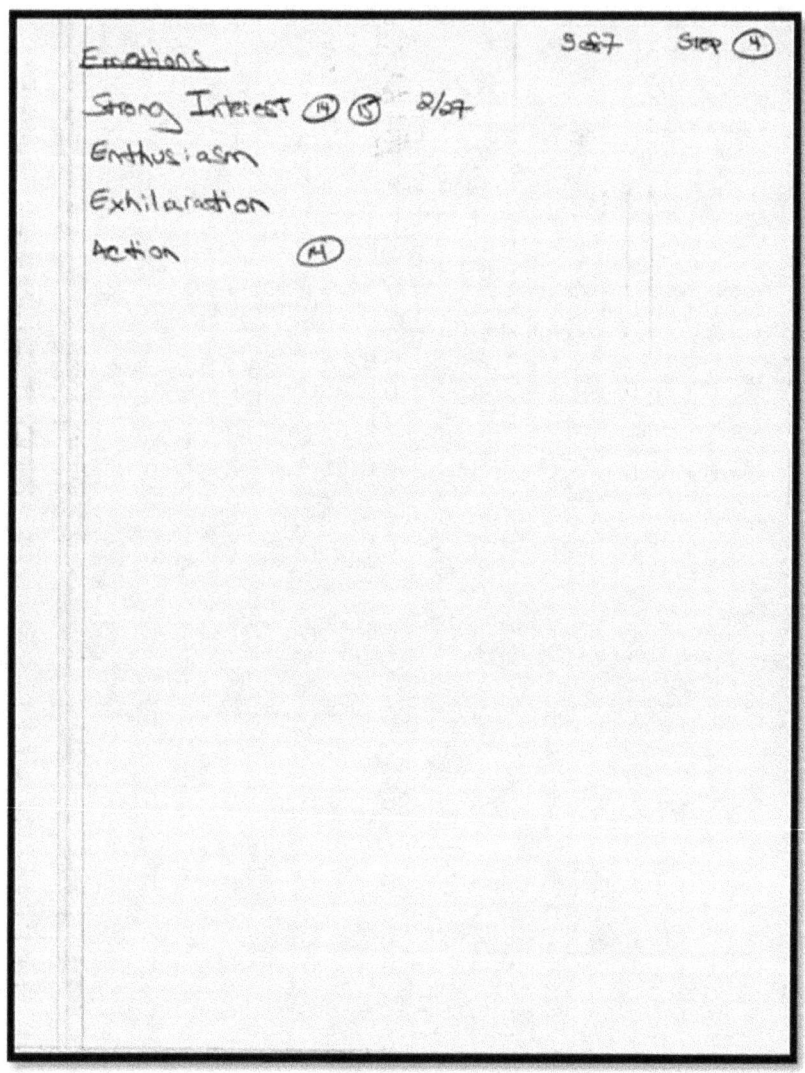

Step 4, 5 of 7

Appendix-A　13

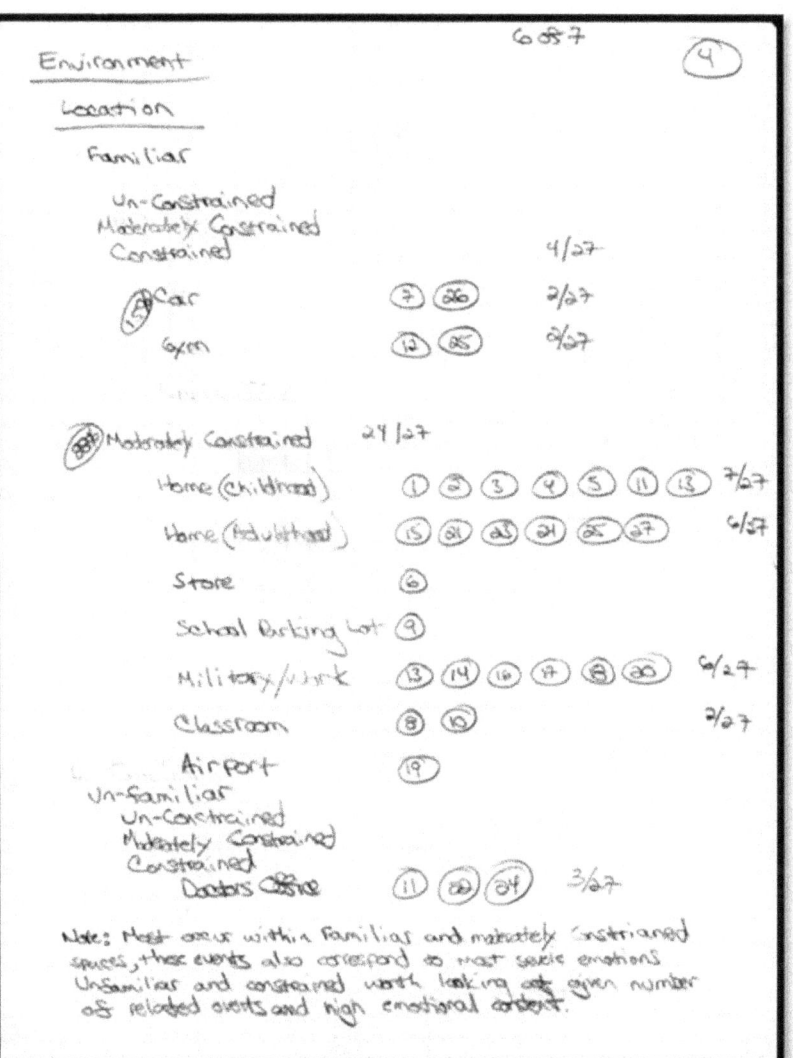

Step 4, 6 of 7

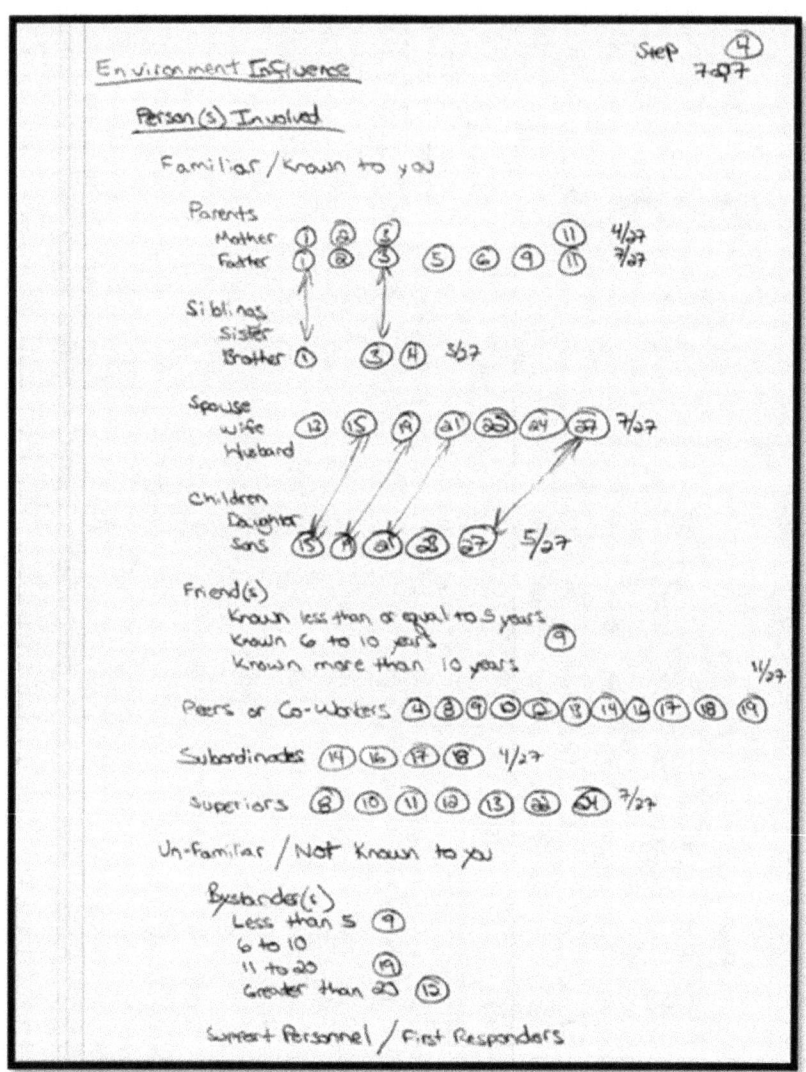

Step 4, 7 of 7

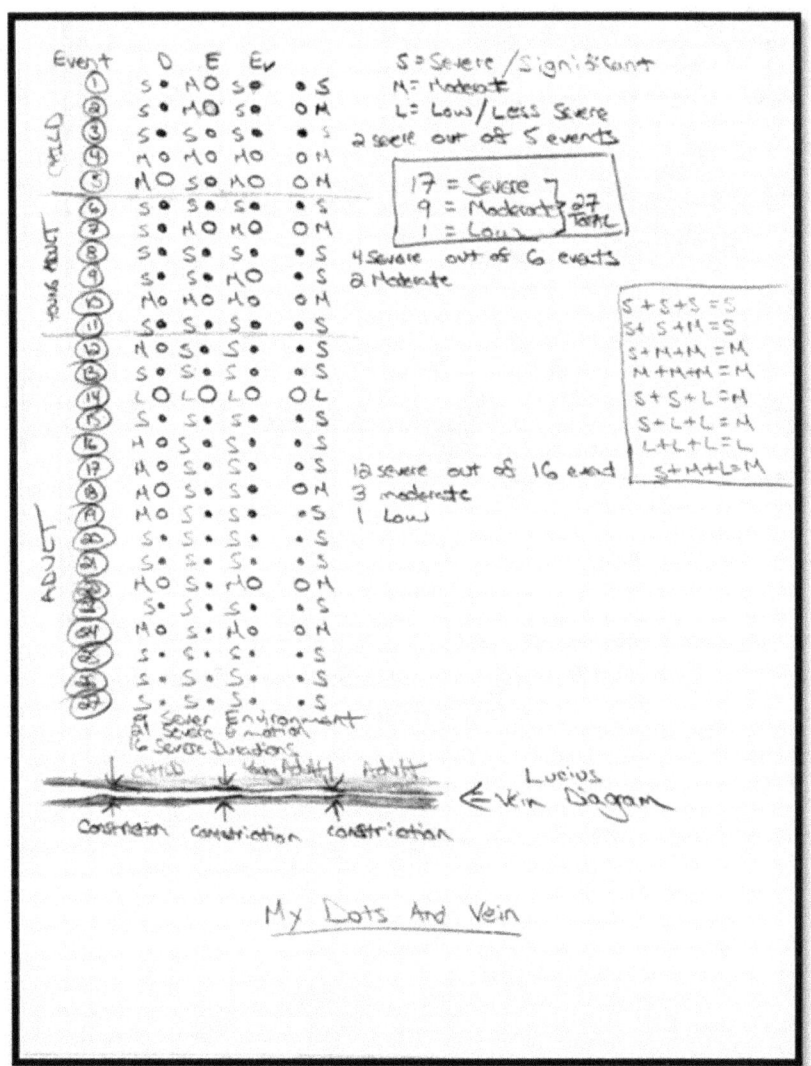

My Seurat Dot's

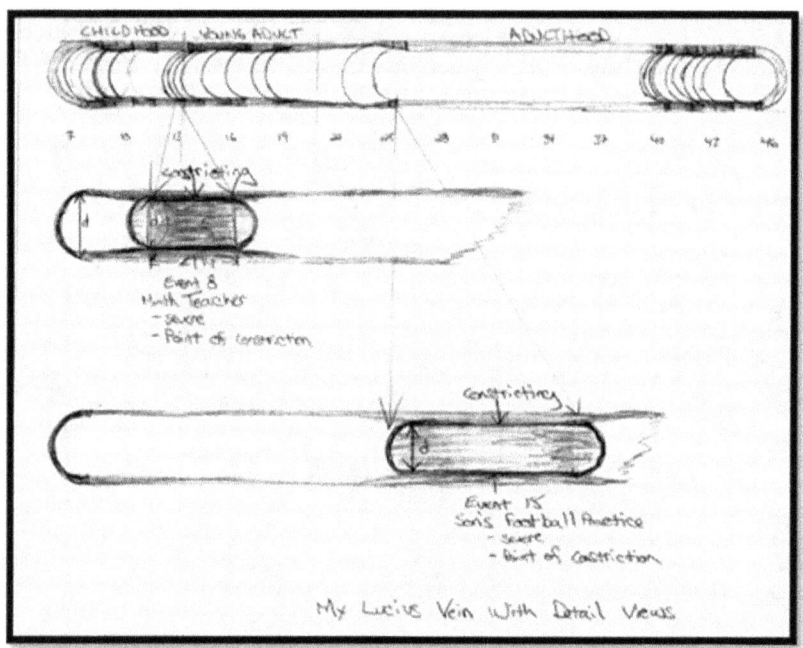

My Lucius Emotional Vein with Details noted from Chronological Experience List

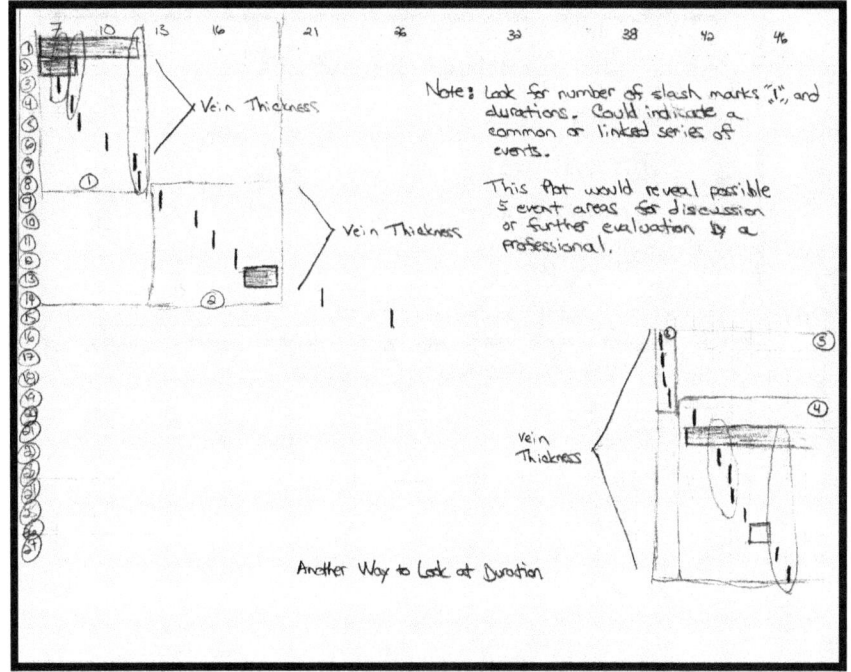

Another way to look at Duration and Time.

- Top Tier Influence Categories
  - Duration
  - Emotion(s)
  - Environment
  - Personality

Influence Categories

serenity of being
postulates
action
exhiliration
aesthetic
enthusiasim
cheerfulness
strong interest
conservative
mild interest
contented
boredom
monotomy
antaganism
hostile
pain
anger
hate
resentment
no sympathy
unexpressed resentment
covert hostility
anxiety
fear
despair
terror
sympathy
propitiation
grief
makingn amends
undeserving
victim
hopeless
failure
pity
blame
regret
dying

Emotions List

Appendix-C   2

- **Environment Influences**
  - **Location**
    - **Rural**
    - **City**
    - **Suburban**
    - **Wooded**
    - **Desert**
    - **Mountainous**
    - **Water**
      - Familiar
        - Confined / Small and enclosed space
        - Moderately Confined / Typical Classroom sized space
        - UN-Confined / Open space
      - Unfamiliar
        - Confined / Small and enclosed space
        - Moderately Confined / Typical Classroom sized space
        - UN-Confined / Open space
      - Environmental Climate Conditions
        - Temperature
          - Severe Heat (greater than 102 degrees F)
          - Hot (85-101 degrees F)
          - Mild (69 -84 degrees F)
          - Cool (52-68 degrees F)
          - Cold (32-51 degrees F)
          - Sever Cold (less than 32 degrees F)
        - Weather Conditions
          - Clear
          - Overcast
          - Light Rain
          - Heavy Rain
          - Light Snow
          - Heavy Snow
          - Sleet
          - Ice
          - Thunder Storm
          - Tropical Storm
          - Hurricane
          - Tornado

Environment Influence (Location)

Appendix-C   3

- **Environment Influence**
  - **People**
    - Familiar
      - Family
        - Immediate
          - Father – Include Step-Father
          - Mother – Include Step-Mother
          - Brother – Include Step-Brother
          - Sister – Include Step-Sister
          - Spouse
            - Husband – Include Ex-Husband
            - Wife – Include Ex-Wife
          - Children / Grand Children
            - Son(s)
            - Daughter(s)
      - Friends
        - Known to you less than 1 year
        - Known to you for more than 1 – 5 years
        - Known to you for more than 6 or more years
      - Peers / Coworkers / Students
      - Superiors
      - Subordinates
    - **Un-Familiar**
      - By Standers
        - Between 1-4
        - Between 5-10
        - Between 11-20
        - Between 21-50
        - More than 51
      - First Responders / EMS

Environment Influence (People)

Appendix-C 4

- Personality Traits
  - Shy / Reserved / Introvert
  - Mild Mannered
  - Outgoing / Extrovert

Personality Traits (Me Factor)

Synopsis

The second book in the series by the author of *A Journey in the Fog of Depression: A Military Officer's Experience*; Discover how he utilizes his ability to define processes in the development of a **game changing**, **step by step model,** that blossoms into a fascinating fresh look deep into our own unique experiences.

Imagine how the serendipitous influences of a Roman philosopher, ordered to commit suicide; A French Post-Impressionist painter who places thousands of small colorful dots on a piece of canvas; And a young boy watching a cartoon, fixated on a single commercial all contribute to the development of a unique method used to discover experiences which contributed to his own depression.

Through a detailed and conversationalist approach, he takes the intangible form of an experience and transforms them into a three dimensional object. Using only pencil, graph paper, and pocket change; he graphically demonstrates each step in detail.

Learn how the young boy turned military officer finds himself sitting in his family room, alone, severely depressed, and contemplating his own suicide muttering the words: "The quickest path to freedom is through any vein in your body." The phrase echoes in his mind, resonating, and haunting him. Carrying him deeper into the fog of his depression.

How did these seemingly disparate events so profoundly influence his Journey with depression? How did he formulate a parallelism with such a dark quote contrasted against a work of art?

A compelling book of hope and a unique dissection of the human experience. Developed for the sole purpose of enhancing today's existing therapies available to our active duty personnel, veterans, and their families suffering the devastating effects of depression.

www.ingramcontent.com/pod-product-compliance
Lightning Source LLC
Chambersburg PA
CBHW051216170526
45166CB00005B/1927